UNF#CK YOUR CUNNILINGUS

How to Give and Receive Tongue-Twisting Oral Sex

DR. FAITH G. HARPER

MICROCOSM PUBLISHING
Portland, Ore

UNFUCK YOUR CUNNILINGUS: How to Give and Receive Tongue-Twisting Oral Sex

Part of the 5 Minute Therapy Series
© Dr. Faith Harper, 2022
First edition © Microcosm Publishing, May 17, 2022
ISBN 9781621064879
This is Microcosm #369
Edited by Lydia Rogue
Design by Joe Biel
Illustrations by Gerta Operaku

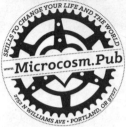

To join the ranks of high-class stores that feature Microcosm titles, talk to your local rep: In the U.S. **COMO** (Atlantic), **FUJII** (Midwest), **BOOK TRAVELERS WEST** (Pacific), **TURNAROUND** (Europe), **UTP/MANDA** (Canada), **NEW SOUTH** (Australia/New Zealand), **GPS** in Asia, Africa, India, South America, and other countries, or **FAIRE** and **NATURE'S RETREAT** in the gift trade.

For a catalog, write or visit:
Microcosm Publishing
2752 N Williams Ave.
Portland, OR 97227
https://microcosm.pub/tongue

Did you know that you can buy our books directly from us at sliding scale rates? Support a small, independent publisher and pay less than Amazon's price at **www.Microcosm.Pub**

Library of Congress Cataloging-in-Publication Data

Names: Harper, Faith G., author.
Title: Unfuck your cunnilingus : how to give and receive tongue-twisting oral sex / Faith G. Harper.
Description: [Portland] : Microcosm Publishing, [2022] | Summary: "Vulvas rejoice! Here is the expert guide you need to the art and science of giving and getting oral pleasure. Learn techniques for causing great pleasure and for communicating desires, needs, and boundaries. Find out the science of why oral sex feels so damn good, work through societal and cultural messages that might get in the way of full enjoyment, and get a good grip on the health, safety, and hygiene stuff you need to know. Dr. Faith G. Harper, sexologist and bestselling author of Unfuck Your Brain and Unfuck Your Intimacy, brings her humor, knowledge, and compassion to help you gain a wonderfully fulfilling sex life"-- Provided by publisher.
Identifiers: LCCN 2021057807 | ISBN 9781621064879 (trade paperback)
Subjects: LCSH: Oral sex. | Sex instruction.
Classification: LCC HQ31.5.O73 H38 2022 | DDC 306.77/4--dc23/eng/20211206
LC record available at https://lccn.loc.gov/2021057807

MICROCOSM·PUBLISHING

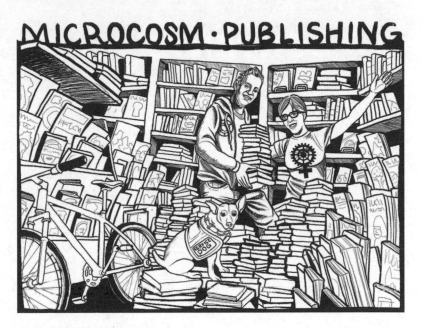

MICROCOSM PUBLISHING is Portland's most diversified publishing house and distributor with a focus on the colorful, authentic, and empowering. Our books and zines have put your power in your hands since 1996, equipping readers to make positive changes in their lives and in the world around them. Microcosm emphasizes skill-building, showing hidden histories, and fostering creativity through challenging conventional publishing wisdom with books and bookettes about DIY skills, food, bicycling, gender, self-care, and social justice. What was once a distro and record label was started by Joe Biel in his bedroom and has become among the oldest independent publishing houses in Portland, OR. We are a politically moderate, centrist publisher in a world that has inched to the right for the past 80 years.

Global labor conditions are bad, and our roots in industrial Cleveland in the 70s and 80s made us appreciate the need to treat workers right. Therefore, our books are MADE IN THE USA.

CONTENTS

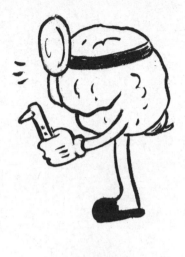
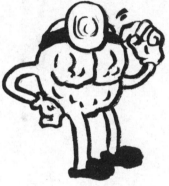
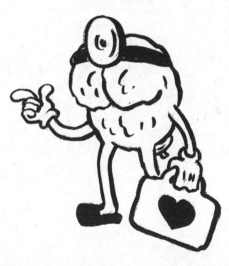

INTRODUCTION

I've written about intimacy in general and boundaries in general. And I've written about sexual consent and sex toys (sex tools!) more specifically. And this book goes in the same pile with those...unfucking our shitty messages about sex and sexuality so you can reclaim your sexual self and make choices that are well-informed, enthusiastic, and freakin' fun.

Cunnilingus is nothing more than oral stimulation of a clitoris.[1] You know, going down. Clam diving. Carpet munching. Eating at the Y. Cunnilingus comes from the Latin words for vulva *(cunnus)* and lick *(lingere)*. So if you are reading this book you may be:

- A person who either provides oral pleasure to a partner with a clitoris (whether one they were born with or one that was bio-constructed) or you are considering adding that to your personal menu.

- You have a clitoris and want to be a better partner when receiving cunnilingus

- You are a research nerd wanting to learn more in general.

I mean, chances are you didn't pick up this book thinking it was about decorating cupcakes. You're here in hopes of learning more about yourself, a current partner(s), potential partner(s), or human peoples in general.

I should also offer caveats that may or may not be obvious. While I am the owner/operator of a vulva, I have not sampled the wares of others. And because I endeavor an approximation of

---

1 Did you know that the plural of clitoris is clitorides?

delivering manuscripts on time, I'm afraid I wouldn't have time to finish this book if I was out on a world-wide tasting menu expedition. So consider this the best advice of a sex educator who has worked diligently to be as inclusive as possible, but definitely is not perfect. And advice contained herein may or may not apply to your real life experiences.

So with all that in mind, let's get started.

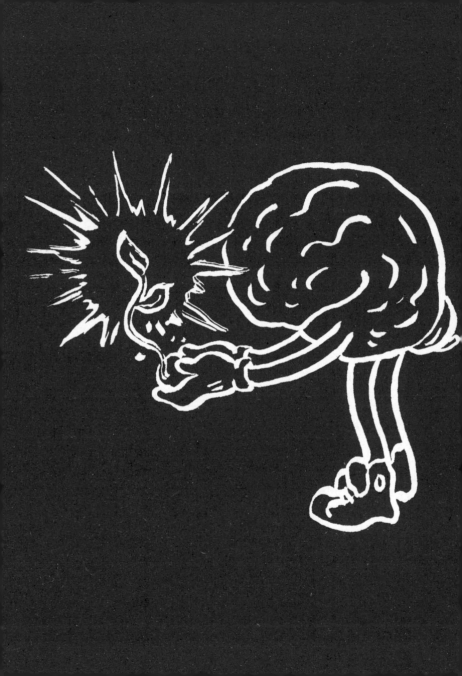

Part One

This Is Your Brain on Cunnilingus

*O*ral sex is kind of a reciprocal trade agreement, when you think about it. It's a negotiation between two (or more) people that is advantageous for everyone involved. Some people like a tongue/mouth (possibly among other things) on their vulva. And some people like to put their tongue/mouth (possibly among other things) on someone else's vulva. And both the receiver and the giver can experience enjoyment, excitement, and fulfillment from the experience.

The word giver is important here. I think the idea that oral sex is purely for the recipient is untrue and part of the shame, stigma, and even mostly-benign snark that surrounds that act. Sex columnist Dan Savage coined the term GGG to mean "good, giving, and game" as a shorthand for the sexual attitudes that are foundational for a healthy sexual relationship. Savage defines GGG as the following: *"Think good in bed, giving based on a partner's sexual interests, and game for anything—within reason."*

This seems reasonable, but is it measurable? Turns out, yes. You won't find research articles that use Savage's verbiage, but you will find a bunch of research on what is termed *sexual transformations*. Sexual transformations[2] are the changes that we make for the sake of our partner or for the relationship itself, meaning *being game*.

Not begrudgingly and eye-rolly but being open to exploring with your partner, in a playful and creative way. Being game means investing your time and energy into something that is an important part of your relationship...and the payoff (sez the researchers) is positive changes in sex, but also other forms of intimacy (cuddling,

---

2 Research nerd alert: This is something that can be conceptualized through a model of dyadic relationships called the actor–partner interdependence model (APIM) which allows for research to be done (like with stats and everything) on the bidirectional effects of relationships.

kissing, etc.), as well as communication and relationship satisfaction in general.

But until pretty far into the 20th century, like the Dr. Faith was alive part of it, oral sex remained something with Roman Empire vibes. In 1950 it was still dead-ass illegal in all 48 states (this was pre Alaska and Hawaii gaining statehood). Likely because of its ties to queer identity.[3] It was something gay men did (e.g., Andy Warhol's movie *Blow Job* (1964) where five different men off screen filated the man on screen). If a straight man received a blow job, it was from a sex worker, not something shared with a GGG partner.

Wanna know who finally got us to shift out of our ancient Roman mindset? The mafia. Seriously.

Mario Puzo's novel "The Godfather" was published in 1969, complete with passages about mutual oral sex between a husband and wife (you know, 69ing). Then the movie adaptation came out in 1972. Additionally, the X rated film *Deep Throat* was shot in January 1972 just a couple of months before *The Godfather* that March (*Deep Throat* released right after in June of the same years). *Deep Throat* was a "blue movie" with a fully realized plot, and it captured national attention and became a cultural touchstone. And? It was financed by members of the Colombo crime family. There is nothing more macho than crime boss shit, right? So as Christopher Hitchens stated in his 2006 *Vanity Fair* piece "As American as Apple Pie" oral sex was "suddenly for real men." It wasn't emasculating to receive or give (!) oral sex.

The mob.

---

3 Keep in mind there were multiple lies criminalizing queerness. The supreme court refused to provide any constitutional protections for oral and anal sex in 1986 (Bowers vs. Hardwick) and it wasn't until Lawrence vs. Texas in 2003 that anal sex was still illegal in 14 states in the U.S.

(Well, and the rise of second wave feminism and a demand for equity in sexual pleasure and orgasms, according to some researchers. But let's go with the mob.)

All of a "sudden," oral sex as part of foreplay and a common part of people's sexual repertoire became increasingly normal. Even for more vanilla couples. By 1994, Kinsey researchers reported that "27% of men and 19% of women have had oral sex in the past year."

By 2012, the CDC published research showing that among 20 to 24 year olds, "81% of females and 80% of males had engaged in oral sex." And even before that (in 2005), another Centers for Disease Control survey on teens and sexual behavior found that young men and women were performing oral sex on each other almost equally. Meaning oral sex isn't just something that is done to and for men. Thank you Mario Puzo for introducing the larger culture to the idea. And then my millennials? Y'all are responsible for the downfall of crappy chain restaurants and the uptick in tongue stuff. And we thank you for your service.

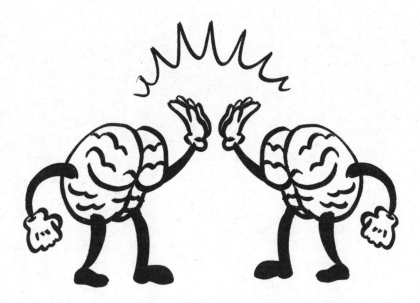

WHY IT FEELS GOOD TO GET CUNNILINGUS

You've probably heard of MRIs (magnetic resonance imaging) which uses magnetic fields and raido waves to create images of tissues and organs and the like. The cool cousin of MRIs are fMRIs (functional magnetic resonance imaging) which indirectly measures neural activity by measuring the patterns and shifts and differences between oxygenated and deoxygenated blood and how it flows in the brain. fMRI research started showing up in the 90s and quickly became the coolest new cognitive neuroscience tool.

It allows brains to be scanned as we are doing stuff, to see how brain regions light up during these activities. No, this doesn't mean "doing X thing caused Y thing in the brain." Correlation isn't causality, but it is incredibly good information and hugely beneficial in figuring out so much of our hows and whys around sex, desire, arousal.

First of all? The best news is that fMRI data backs up the fact that sex is not addictive in the clinical sense of the word. The American Psychiatric Association (the group of people who look at all the science and determine when there is rigorous enough research for something to be classified as a diagnoses that goes in the DSM) is very specific about what constitutes an addiction. Addictions don't just cause intense cravings, imaging researchers have demonstrated that they *change* personalities, behaviors, our ability to learn and retain what we learned, and how we move our bodies. These are usually caused by substances, which cause significant changes in not just how the brain functions but how it's structured. Only one non-substance causes these same levels of changes, and that is gambling. Not sex.

This doesn't mean that we can't have out of control behaviors about most anything. You have probably done dumb shit that felt very out of control. If not around sex, around something. Sex tends to be a big one though. Because everyone's brains light up during sex. *They are supposed to.*

Even though there are physiological differences in how we orgasm based on our sex assigned at birth, how our brains react are exactly the same. And there is no "sexual center" of the brain, there are more than thirty system areas that become engaged. Our touch processing centers getting activated clearly makes sense. But other "seemingly unrelated" areas like the memory and emotions part (limbic system), the body movement part (the hypothalamus), and the judgment and problem solving part (the prefrontal cortex) all have things to say.

The hypothalamus works to quickly produce oxytocin that assists with enhanced arousal. The logical part (the lateral orbitofrontal cortex) dials way down, in order to dispel normal fear and anxiety about vulnerability while the limbic system pulls up are previous associations with movment and touch and memories about other sexual encounters. This is why, yes, those of us who have trauma histories can struggle to relax into sex regardless of whether or not the initial trauma was sexual.

We also activate a bunch of hormones and neurochemicals. The big ones are oxytocin (which is a bonding/attachment/social safety hormone). And dopamine (pleasure, desire, and motivation). And for my people who are thinking "Hah! Dopamine! Addictive!"

it's important to realize that these chemicals and chemical pathways light up during sex and orgasm, not in similar ways to that of a drug, but in very similar ways to other normal, human pleasurable experiences. Like listening to your favorite song or eating your favorite meal.

Delight is not addiction.

Further, regular orgasms have been correlated with good health outcomes. The prevailing idea is that the extra brain activity and consistent blood flow activation to those regions of the brain.

So why oral in particular?

If you ask 1,000 different people, you will get 1,000 different answers as to why they like what they like. Some people like oral sex way better than any other kind of sex, some think of it as a fun part of diverse menu but maybe not their favorite thing, and some people are just not that into it.

Some people are unable to, for a multitude of reasons, engage in penatrative intercourse and oral sex allows them to imtimately connect with a partner.

Some like that it feels like penetrative intercourse, specifically hot and wet. It may not feel as tight as penetration, but there is the added option of creating light suction instead which can feel great for some people.

Others love the opportunity to be taken care of, the vulnerability of doing so, and being able to focus on enjoying their own pleasure.

Still others like the sounds or the visuals of it. The wet slurping sounds, the humming, and other noises. And the aesthetics of being able to see what's happening in a different way. You are generally positioned in such a way that you can watch your partner engaging in something for your pleasure, which has been described as being akin to watching yourself star in your own erotic performance venture.

And if none of these apply to you? Feel free to mentally insert your own.

WHY WE LIKE TO GIVE CUNNILINGUS

*T*he biggest, realest answer as to why we like to give our partners oral?

It's fun.

Pleasing our partners is fun. Their pleasure can provide us pleasure. Sex is supposed to be an enjoyable thing, so there ya go.

What else?

Going back again to the individuals that cannot have penetrative intercourse or are choosing not to? Oral sex gets centered as our means of partnered sexual expression. Penetrative intercourse, especially the presumed penis-in-vagina kind, doesn't have to be centered as the "proper way to have sex." And isn't it fun to have something else from the sexual menu? And defy all cultural expectations of how we are supposed to have sex?

Anything else? For those of you who want something more science-y or you will be disappointed in my academic database research skills? There actually *is* a possible evolutionary explanation. Authors of a 2010 article published in *Journal of Reproductive Immunology* point out that a multitude of pregnancy problems have been correlated with the pregnant parent's body rejecting the other parent's genes as foreign. The idea, then, is that swallowing the semen of your partner helps your body become accustomed to your partner's DNA thus making it less likely for you to reject their sperm should y'all end up baby-making.

Another study, this one published in *Evolutionary Psychology*, found that when someone perceives their partner as being a "get" (meaning they have competition), are more likely to perform oral sex on their partner to keep them satisfied/less likely to wander off with the competition. The authors of this article, speaking specifically to monogamous heterosexual cisgender couples, posit that it makes it much more likely for men to pass on their genes if the woman in question doesn't leave him for someone who is better at pleasing them.

So sure, maybe. There could totally be some evolutionary benefits to oral sex. Though why things evolved to happen and why we do them now are not necessarily related. Especially since most of us are not in such relationship configurations. "Because it feels good" is a perfectly valid reason to do something.

WHEN THINGS DON'T WORK FANTASTICALLY

*T*he term of *sexual dysfunction* is an umbrella term used to refer to any problem anywhere in the sexual response cycle (motivation/desire, arousal, orgasm, resolution) that impedes our pleasure. Issues that fall in this category include:

- Anorgasmia: Inability to have an orgasm

- Dyspareunia: Experiencing pain during sex

- Hypoactive sexual desire disorder: Lack of desire or libido

- Sexual arousal disorder: Problems with arousal

Research demonstrates that one or more of these issues affects about 30% to 40% of individuals with vaginas and vulvas, with low desire levels being most common. But as history has consistently shown regarding medical understanding of our bodies, there are some likely accuracy problems with these numbers.

Most of the arousal research has focused on genital congestion (blood rushing to the area and erectile tissue becoming erect) and lubrication, because that has typically been a good measure for individuals with penes. But sexual excitement for us starts with thoughts and emotions. It's far more subjective than just a measure of vasocongestion.[4]

Additionally, we are less likely to experience spontaneous desire and spontaneous sexual fantasies, and are more likely to

4 It's dark, but fascinating research. People with vaginas and vulvas will respond to sexual stimuli even if they aren't psychologically turned on…when individuals with penes will not. It's thought to be an evolutionary protective mechanism since we, during the course of human history, have not had a whole lot of say in sexual partners and activities. It's an adaptation to prevent damage from things being *done to us*.

experience our sexual selves as a part of ourselves we connect to, draw forth, and share with a partner (Esther Perel's book *Mating in Captivity* speaks to this further).

The other common human experience is low libido. Libido exists on a spectrum. Not just among different people but even within ourselves. Low libido (aka hyposexual sexual desire disorder, impaired sexual function, diminished sex drive, etc) is the mind-willing part of sexual expression. It's about the *wanting* to have sex, versus the physical excitement around sex (like an erection or lack thereof). The Mayo Clinic notes these signs of low libido:

- Loss of interest in any form of sexual activity, both partnered and solo

- Lack of sexual fantasies or thoughts

- Feeling unhappy or worried about either or both of the above

This is a well thought out list of indicators because it really focuses on something changing in a way that is not perceived as for the better. It also accounts for someone who is asexual, greysexual, or demisexual. But if it's you and you're miserable about it? It could be the result of many different things. Stress, drug and alcohol usage, not sleeping for shit, other physical and mental health conditions (hormonal changes being a big one), toxin exposure, relationship stressors. One of the other big culprits for low libido is medications, both over the counter and prescription. The medications that may cause these conditions are listed below, because that's the easiest fix in the bunch. Speaking to your doctor about changing up your medications may resolve the issue quickly. But if that doesn't do the trick, we are going into a lot of other strategies later in the book that may help, as well.

Other health issues that can harsh our mellow include:

- Hormonal changes (which can lead to vaginal dryness and even atrophy, which makes penetrative intercourse particularly painful, but all kinds of sex may also be unfun)

- Medical conditions that affect the vagina/vulva directly like endometriosis, ovarian cysts, uterine fibroids, vaginal inflammation (vaginitis), and vaginal muscle spasms (vaginismus). Interestingly enough, most of the testosterone women produce is in our ovaries, so ovarian production of testosterone getting shut down

- Vascular issues (anything that affects blood flow, particularly to the vagina/vulva/labia/clitoris)

- Other health conditions (diabetes, heart disease, high blood pressure, multiple sclerosis, arthritis, and anything that affects pain and mobility)

- Medications and treatments (chemotherapy, other cancer treatments, and many types of antidepressants are the biggest culprits but not the only ones)

- Depression (depression is a total libido killer....50% of the individuals that struggle with major depressive disorder have sex drive, sex arousal, and even vaginal lubrication issues), stress levels (cortisol decreases sex drive), drug/alcohol addiction, trauma history (especially related to physical sexual abuse)

- Toxin exposure (ugh, the inflammation)

- Sleep disorders
- A stationary lifestyle (bodies really need to move, and if that isn't part of our regular daily activities, including getting exercise, they get grumpy)
- Body image and self-consciousness
- Relationship problems in general

MEDICATIONS THAT CAN LEAD TO LOW LIBIDO
Prescription Medications:

- Anti-anxiety medications based on benzodiazepines (Xanax)
- Anticonvulsant medications (such as, Tegretol, Phenytoin, Phenobarbital)
- Antidepressants (including, anti-mania medications, antipsychotics, MAOIs, SSRIs, SNRIs, tricyclic antidepressants)
- Benign prostatic hyperplasia treatments (such as Flomax, Propecia, Proscar)
- Cancer treatments (including radiation and chemotherapy)
- Heart and blood pressure medications (including, ACE inhibitors, a-Adrenergic blockers, b-adrenergic (beta) blockers, centrally acting agents, diuretics, thiazides, and statins)
- Hormonal contraceptives (such as Ortho Tri-Cyclen)
- Opioid pain relievers (such as Vicodin, Oxycontin, and Percocet)

- Steroid medications (including anabolic steroids and corticosteroids)

Over-the-counter medications:

- Antifungals, specifically ketoconazole or fluconazole

- Antihistamines, including Benadryl (diphenhydramine) and Chlor-Trimeton (chlorpheniramine)

- Tagamet (cimetidine)

Recreational Drugs:

This category is harder to listicle, because people's experiences of them vary widely. Alcohol and THC are examples of super-common substances that elevate libido in some people and crash it out in others. So anything you are taking may be having a frustrating impact on your sex life.

All medications operate in the body differently. Time to take effect and time to clear out. So not taking it for one day may or may not be an efficacious litmus test. Read up on whatever you're taking and talk to your prescriber about anything that they have given you. What are options for titrating your dosage or stopping altogether? Can this be done safely? What other side effects might occur that you need to watch for? When would you notice a difference? All that complicated adult-y stuff

Age-related Changes

Oh, my bouncing baby Buddha, save us from the idea that our sexual primes are in our twenties. And praise be sex therapist David Schnarch, author of the book *Passionate Marriage* for challenging the notion by pointing out that there's a big different between one's genital prime and one's sexual prime

Sure, our genital primes (the physicality of how our bodies function) are when we are younger. But our sexual primes? Not until way later. A study of men in Norway found that those in their 50s experienced more sexual satisfaction than they did in their 30s, even if not everything is as hard, wet, or quick to bounce back, or whatever else we may miss from our youth.

As we get older and have had more sex, we leave behind our exploratory years and enter the years of self-confidence. We know what we like. We know how we like it. We are exhausted of the insecurities that the larger culture has foisted upon us and we started living to be comfortable in our bodies. Which leads to better sexual encounters and orgasms. And if you feel that you aren't there yet? You're literally doing the research to help you get there, which makes you a total badass.

And yes, older generations are still having lots of sex. Even generations that came of age pre-sexual revolution.[5] Because bodies do age and like to do wonky, non-behaving things sometimes, oral sex can become an even more integral part of sexual connection with a partner (read: penetrative intercourse can become more difficult to accomplish for a multitude of reasons). Many older couples related oral sex to a better quality of relationship and overall life happiness than younger people do in studies on sexual behavior.

---

5 Specifics? Got you, boo. A study of 884 heterosexual couples from the National Social Life, Health, and Aging Project in 2010 found that more than half of those aged 57 to 75 said they engaged in oral sex as did about a third of 75- to 85-year-olds.

Due to Disability

Disabilities can be something we are born with (genetic) or something that can happen to us at any time (acquired). In both cases, there may be fuckery to overcome beyond living in a body that isn't performing the way you want it to. The cultural messages around disability (and the presumption that you now exist in the category of non-sexual), are slowly changing, though we still have a long way to go.

Later in this book we are going to get more granular about adaptations that can help you better enjoy your sexual self, but for right here I think it's most important to note that while individuals with physical disabilities report engaging in mutual sexual activity less frequently than able-bodied folks (especially for folks who struggle with day-to-day tasks without assistance/support), there are many things that predict sexual satisfaction and sexual esteem.

Additionally, the longer we live with the physical limitations of our bodies, the more positive we feel about ourselves as sexual beings. Just like we feel more comfortable with our sexual selves as we get older, we also have the capacity to grow into a level of comfort with our bodies over time as well. Partnered sexual activity focuses more on other parts of the menu and one of the things most frequently mentioned is oral sex.

Which is to say, oral sex is a solution, not the problem.

While on Hormone Therapy

Despite what a neoconservative politician would have you believe, most of the people on hormone therapy are *not* doing so as part of gender affirmative care. Meaning most people on hormones are cisgender. For some people, hormone therapy can be a game changer in terms of desire, arousal, and performance. But because the brain is the biggest sex organ in the human body, our self-concept also has a huge impact on our sexual desire. The entirety of our bodies change with hormones and someone being on hormones for a thyroid condition, as an example, may not feel great about how that changes their physical appearance which can in turn affect arousal.

Additionally? Someone who is on the trans spectrum, and is on a hormone therapy regimen as part of their care, may also notice changes in their arousal patterns and changes in how they perceive their body which impacts sexual desire just as much as it can for a cis person.

Even if you are loving all of the health benefits of hormone therapy, you may find that your erogenous zones have changed which is something important to communicate with a partner.

Part Two

How Our Cunnilingus Gets Fucked Up

$\mathcal{W}$ell, it wouldn't be a Dr. Faith book if we didn't start with how we get fucked up, right? The fuckery. If you have struggled with this, or felt anxious, or uncomfortable and not sure why? We might just be able to unravel some of that together.

External Factors and Stigmas

Sex is super important to most people. Not everyone (I see you my sex-repulsed and sex-neutral peeps), but most everyone. While old cranks and media pontificators like to rail about how modern culture has permissioned us to be sex obsessed freaks, that's dead-ass not true. Human beings always HAVE been sex-obsessed freaks.

Humans invented the dildo before the wheel. Not just a few years before the wheel, but *25,000 years* before the wheel.

Priorities.

The original dildos were made out of stone (ok, makes sense) and other materials like dried camel dung (please, please don't). But that's not all. It was super openly discussed and shared. Sex and sexy toy usage was depicted in cave paintings . . . going back to paleolithic cave art. Our earliest ancestors were as kinky as we are, bless their hearts.

In his book *Ethical Porn For Dicks*, Dr. David Ley refers to these early images as "petro-porn" (love that) and also points out that these images not only exist across all human cultures, they were also placed in areas where the light of the campfire would cast shadows that would turn the still images into flickering stop-motion mini-movies.

Cunnilingus was not a dirty thing early in human history. In fact, it was revered. For example, the earliest known civilization… Sumeria (the area now part of modern day Iraq) was very pro-yummy of oral sex. There was a Sumerian lovesong (this is like 2000 BCE mind you) that translates to *Like her mouth her vulva is sweet, like her vulva her mouth is sweet*. And Taoists of ancient China promoted ingesting the vaginal secretions of one's partner in order to strengthen their own Yang.

In case you are looking for a new religion or anything.

And in the common era, the *Kama Sutra* did not once stutter in its insistence that men should give women orgasms. In fact the Sanskrit word for clitoris is smara-chattra which means *umbrella to the god of love*.

In case you are looking for a new band name or anything.

But because we clearly are not allowed to have nice things for long, things started going dark during the Hellenistic period.[6] Cunnilingus started getting made fun of/dismissed as something only lesbians or men who can't get an erection do.

Then the Romans said "hahaha, hold my mead" and went on to dictate that the word clitoris (landīca) is an obscenity. The actual appropriate word for the body part became as not-OK as the word cunt, and started only showing up in graffiti.

Then? The fall of the Roman Empire actually made things worse. It led to a lot of seperatist feudal kingdoms, weirdly segregated populations, and a spread of different sects of Christianity. And? Long-story-short? This also spread

6 The era of Mediterranean culture that occured after the death of Alexander the Great (323 BC) and the beginning of the Roman empire (31 BC).

new weird rules about sexual acts. Yes, sects killed sex. As certain cultural paradigms changed, criminalization of human sexuality increasingly became the norm. We know that these practices still happened because *most humans have sex*. But ways of experiencing and sharing pleasure that did not relate directly to procreation become increasingly punished (sound familiar?).

Although of course, no one stopped doing fun stuff. And documentation still demonstrates the ubiquity of human sexual expression in all its various forms. After spending time being relegated to graffiti, it started appearing in documents that are referred to by historians as *penitential literature,* documents related to punishments or penances owed for these ridiculous forms of sex that were being done for FUN instead of BABY MAKING. For example, one document from Ireland, specially decreed four years of penance for cunnilingus (and seven years for repeat offenders for cunnilingus, in case you wondered.)

But if that wasn't dark enough, we moved into treating oral sex from something kinda chafa into something that was considered downright evil. The women's holocaust, the witch trials of Europe and then the colonies, fucked us up but good for a very long time. A 15th century witch hunting guide referred to clitorides as the devil's teat. Meaning its mere existence made one a witch. Then there are trial records from Massachusetts that contain explicit information regarding both cunnilingus and female ejaculate as evidence of witchcraft that led the defendant to be put to death.

Hundreds of years of these kinds of laws (which still exist in some areas) and continued struggle with this level of purity culture has created a complicated glop of ideas to unfuck. What we think

we are *supposed* to like and what we *actually* like are competing
ideas, even to this day.

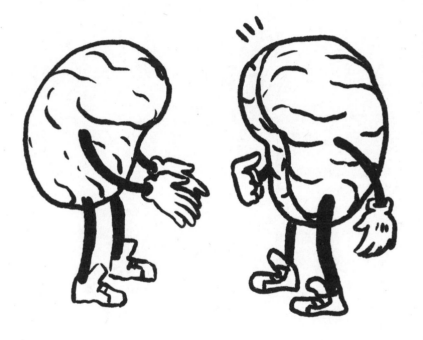

INTERNALIZED CUNNILINGUS FUCKENING

*A*s you might expect, alot of our internalized issues with oral sex started with these larger cultural messages discussed above.

But *then*.

We add in our over-worried, over-thinkied, over-anxious brains to the mix and while we may have moved past larger social messages, we still struggle with our own sense of enough-ness.

Meaning, we think other people deserve fun and healthy sex lives, but not us. We're gross. We look weird, we smell weird, no one wants to put their face....you know....down THERE. Most people are aware there is a good amount of research on body image in general, but genital self-image is prevalent enough also to have been studied scientifically. Zero surprise in that how we feel about our bodies overall and our genitalia in particular changes our overall sexual experiences.

Another huge issue for many people is their trauma history. Unresolved trauma, by definition, involves numbness/avoidance followed by hyper arousal and reactivity. Meaning not feeling anything and then feeling too much. And the feeling too much is related to the previous trauma, not current events. And many traumatic events (not just sexual assault, abuse, and rape) are heavily somatic, meaning they create huge swings when it comes to desire, arousal, and orgasm. This can look like being hyposexual or hypersexual, and even moving quickly between the two states regularly.

Masters and Johnson researchers pointed out back in the 1990s (in a study published by the US Department of Justice!!), that the dissociation (disembodiment) that often appears regularly among individuals with trauma histories can be incredibly common in mediating sexual expression. The ability to detach, important to trauma survival, can continue to kick in regularly in our lives. And many people will continue to have sex from this place of detachment, so the physiology of of our bodies is still online but not our emotional states. This allows us to shut off the "this person may be dangerous" part of our brain but also "this is a partner with whom I choose to have a connection" part as well, which definitely can end up being a problem.

All of this is to say, if you notice that you struggle with intimacy, oscillate back and forth on feeling connected and disconnected (with nothing different going on with that partner), or find that it's all fine as long as you are thinking about something else? These may be trauma reactions. And you deserve to heal what is unhealed in you, not just for your sex life but for all aspects of your life.

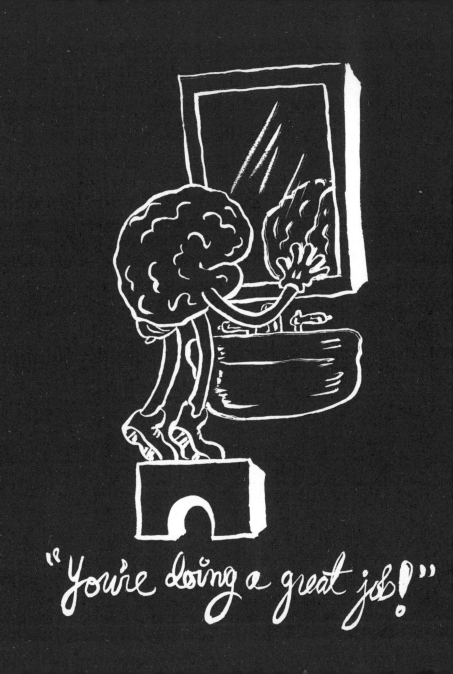

"You're doing a great job!"

Part Three

Unfuck Your Cunnilingus

So if any of this resonates, you are not alone. But the good news? One of my favorite grad school professors once pointed out to me that culture is *anything we create*. We. Me and you. Out there changing the word for ourselves and other people. Let's create a culture in which we get to enjoy what we enjoy and tap out of things we don't with no hard feelings, yeah?

There is no way to talk about it without just talking about it. Just like the only way out of Mordor is through Mordor. Uncomfortable, whether or not y'all are brand new or been together a minute. Though as uncomfortable as it feels, it becomes far easier and more natural with very little time. It's totally ok to throw me under the bus and say "So I'm reading this book that has more information about oral sex than I thought existed on the planet. While she probably takes the whole topic way too seriously, I did realize we never have discussed what we like and don't like in that regard."

Because with very few exceptions, your partner is going to know their body way better than you do. And the resounding theme of the rest of this chapter is "Here is an idea….if you and your partner are into it." Meaning, every body operates differently and there is no one right way to give head.

Ok, I take that back, there is. The one right way to give head is to communicate clearly with your partner and then enjoy the agreed-upon plan together.

Other than admitting you were reading this book, how else can you open up the conversation? A lot of my couple-clients (and throuple and so on FWIW) have found using a yes/no/maybe checklist as a solid way of opening up the conversation. But before we even do that, a lot of peeps also really benefit from a from starting with an identity conversation. Not just the "my name is [blank] and my pronouns are [blank]" but getting even more specific to how that relates to their body and their sexual expression. This format is one I modified from a yes/no/maybe checklist written by Tab Kimpton as part of the Khaos Komix series.

Identity Information

- I describe my gender as:

- My pronouns are:

- My gender descriptor words are: (femme, butch, boi)

- My sexual orientation identity words are:

- My sexual role (e.g. top, bottom) words are:

- My terms for my chest/breasts are:

- My terms for my genitals are:

- My terms for my prostate/Gräfenberg spot are:

- My terms for my anal region/alimentary canal are:

- These terms are:

____ relatively static for me

____ regularly fluid for me.

- If I am fluid, this is how I communicate that information to a partner so they know to shift language:

- Some words I am not okay with to refer to me, my identity, my body or, or which I am uncomfortable using or hearing are:

- I am activated (and not in a good way) by certain words or language. Those are/that is:

- Are certain words okay in some settings or situations but not in others?

- How so? (Explanation not required unless you want to, just which situations should be watched for)

- How flexible am I with what a partner might want to call something I like calling something else?

- Any other important information to share?

Yes/No/Maybe Checklists

Great! Next helpful part? Sharing with a partner/partners what you're into. These checklists can be super intricate, involved, and intensive and many of my clients have reported back "Ok, so I'm not kinky at all, considering all the possibilities out there." So trying to create an inclusive one here is pretty impossible. Also, there are really good ones already available, including ones that are more specific to different interests and one that is designed specifically for visual communicators. Some are more specific than others. One is better for visual thinkers and the last one on the list is specific for consensual non-monogamy. Check them out online and see if any feel like a good starting place for you:

- Sexual Interests Checklist (AskingForWhatYouWant. com)

- Yes/No/Maybe List (SexWithEmily.com)

- Yes, No, Maybe So: A Sexual Inventory Stocklist (Scarleteen.com)

- The Super Powered Yes/No/Maybe List: A Negotiation Tool for Sex Nerds (BexTalksSex.com)

- Navigating Consent & Setting Sexual Boundaries: Yes/No/Maybe List (SunnyMegatron.com)

- You Need Help: Here Is A Worksheet To Help You Talk To Partners About Sex: A List For Visual People (Autostraddle.com)

- Poly Yes/No/Maybe List (Polynotes.tumblr.com)

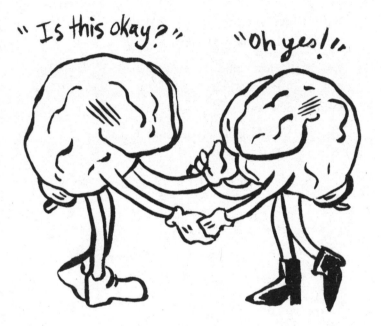

CONSENT

Consent is the informed, voluntary agreement reached for an activity/exchange between two or more sentient beings. When it comes to the expression and negotiation of our boundaries, we generally do so through how we communicate consent. At its most basic level, consent is permission for something to happen. And most importantly, our permission should be punctuated with an exclamation point. In an ideal situation, you aren't having to be convinced, you're saying "yes!" Consent provides a safe framework for interactions. For those of us with trauma histories, a safe framework can be a very healing experience. And, equally important, it allows us to experience own our desires in a sex-positive way.

Permissive consent is what allows us to engage in specific actions in relation to those cultural standards of practice and social norms. For example, originating consent holds that it is not acceptable behavior to stab needles into another human being on the regular, right? But if you go see a tattoo artist, sign their waiver, and pay them for their work, you are engaging in permissive consent.

Permissive consent is our expression of boundaries in context. And despite all our conversations about active, continuous consent the reality is that most consent is not verbal. This isn't good or bad, it's just something to be aware of.

Permissive consent is established in one of three ways:

Explicit Consent: Explicit consent requires the "yes" to be spoken. It is directly expressed consent. A contract that is reviewed, understood, and signed before any exchange is explicit consent. Asking another person "may I____your____" is explicit consent. When we talk about active, continuous consent (meaning active agreement to activity with continued check-ins that the activity is still a go) we are talking about explicit consent.

Implicit Consent: Implicit consent operates on presumptions of nos and yeses. It is the inference of consent based on our actions and circumstances. This isn't a fundamentally terrible thing. We do it all the time. If I purchase a bag of pistachios and leave it on my husband's desk, the implication is that they are there for him to eat. If you apply for a job and your resume includes the names and contact information for references, the implication is that the potential employer will call them to verify your employment eligibility. This is also the area that gets people in the most trouble, such as when someone presumes that engaging in one sexual activity implies consent for another activity that wasn't discussed.

Blanket/Opt-Out/Meta-Consent: These types of consent require a "no" to be spoken. They give the opportunity for the no and if the no is not forthcoming, the "yes" is presumed. This is another common way of operating within close relationships. For example, someone you know well may hug you when they see you and the presumption would be that that is a norm in your relationship. If you weren't down for a hug, you would say "I'm super touched out today, I need a mulligan on the hug" to let them know there was a change in your normal interactions. An example within the BDSM community would be in edge play, where the dom is setting the scene but the sub has a safeword that they can invoke.

Consent is foundational. Healthy behaviors cannot exist without consent being the first part of the equation. But the minute we start saying "I, too, have a personhood to be respected" through the act of establishing and communicating boundaries, we are changing our relationships and our expectations of interactions within our surrounding community. We are evolving toward equity in interaction for the betterment of all humans.

Sample Consent Contract

Since our contemporary conversation around consent started within the kink community, let's look at one of the more formal consent tools that has come from the aforementioned community. Some people may snicker at the idea, but a written consent contract doesn't exist for the purpose of earning extra-woke brownie points. They make sense for BDSM play, but even beyond that, they create a foundation and structure for a conversation about active, continuous consent. And that's not woke-ness...that's badass, thoughtful adulting.

I, _____, hereby declare under penalty of perjury that I am over 18 years old and am not under the influence of intoxicants or medications that inhibit my ability to affirm consent.

I further declare that this agreement is of my own free will and that neither I nor anyone near or dear to me has been threatened with negative consequences if I chose not to enter into this contract.

Both parties agree that this is a private agreement not to be disclosed to third parties except in case of accusation of sexual misconduct by an agreeing party.

If an agreeing party shows or makes public this agreement without accusation of sexual misconduct, it is agreed that they will be liable for damages for invasion of privacy.

By initialing, _____ I agree to engage in all or some of the following consensual acts.

_____

With the following individual(s)

_____

Safer sex methods that I want utilized during these acts include:

_____

At this time I do not intend to change my mind before the sex act or acts are over. However, if I do, it is further understood that when I say the words _____ or make the signal (hand gesture, etc.) _____ all involved parties/partners agree to STOP INSTANTLY!

Signed:_____Date:_____

Signed: _____ Date: _____

Disclaimer: This sample contract does not constitute legal advice and is provided for educational purposes only. Check with legal counsel before entering into any agreement.

But What If I Don't Know Enough About Myself To Know What Turns Me On?

As frustrating as it feels to be in a situation where you don't know what gets your engines revved, please know that you are far from alone and you are miles away from unusual. We think of sexual desire as something that someone gives us. That is, it's someone's job to turn us on.

That's an oversimplification of how *contextual* desire really is.

In reality, our sexual expression comes from something within us that we, in turn, can choose to share with a partner. Rosemary Basson's sexual desire model[7] demonstrates that there are several steps that we get to that are about our internal world and our connection to our erotic selves before we get to actual sexual desire.

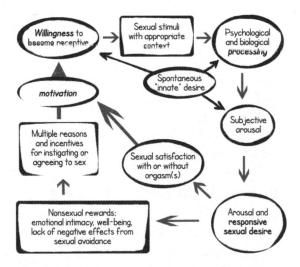

---

7 Dr. Basson's model is an explanation of the sexual excitement cycle of cis women. And while there are absolutely differences among the genders and just within humans in general, I've found that mindset and self-knowledge is important to everyone.

While expanding our repertoire and trying new things and experimentation is also a fun part of being a sexual being, so is slowing down and connecting back to ourselves and what we like and don't like. It's another form of mindfulness. It means being curious within ourselves instead of judgemental. And letting go of the rules and assumptions we have created for ourselves and our sexual encounters.

This all ties to consent as a continuous process, that requires us to listen in to our own bodies just as a continuously. What was right for you in the past and what may be right for you in the future, may not serve you in the present.

Let's look at some questions to help you connect to that space:

1) When did you feel like your most authentic self (connected and grounded in your body)?

2) What things were you doing for yourself that helped facilitate that?

3) What activities give you energy or feel worth the energy they take?

4) What activities feel playful to you?

5) What gets you curious and interested in life?

Engagement Through the 5 Senses

Another way we can build a solid understanding of how we connect to our inner eroticism is by understanding how we most strongly engage in the world. We all explore the world through our 5 senses (or at least as many of these senses as we have access to) and we all tend to be more strongly engaged through one or two of the than the others. In her book *Urban Tantra: Sacred Sex for the Twenty-First Century*, Barbara Carrellas points out that recognizing which sense we most connect to can help us receive with more intentionality. So let's look at where you stand, yeah?

VISUAL
When you recall details about an event do you most easily go to what you saw? How easily can you visualize your childhood home? Where you live now? What your favorite person looks like? Is how someone looks or how they move their body sensual to you?

KINESTHETIC
When you recall details about an event do you most easily remember how things felt when you engaged them with your body? How easily can you remember what your favorite article of clothing feels like on your skin? Picking up a warm mug when your hands are cold? The sensation of jumping into a pool of water? What a partner's body feels like when it connects with yours?

AUDITORY
When you recall details about an event do you most easily remember what you heard other people say or noises that were made? How easily can you remember someone's tone of voice? How easily do you learn and retain information when it is told to you verbally? Do you most connect with the sounds a partner makes during sex?

OLFACTORY

When you recall details about an event do you most easily remember what things smelled like? How easily can you remember what your elementary school classroom smelled like? Your favorite flower? Your favorite perfume or cologne? Do you most connect to a partner's scent?

GUSTATORY

When you recall details about an event do you most easily remember what things tasted like? Can you easily recall the taste and texture of your favorite food? Can you see or hear about something and imagine what it would taste like immediately? Do you most connect with how your partner tastes when you kiss or lick them?

If you are noticing some clear differences in how quickly and clearly certain memories come up based on one of two of your senses, this can provide some great cues on how you connect to your own sexual desire and how you share that with a partner. Practice engaging the world with these senses more on a daily basis and more with a partner and see what new things you start to figure out about yourself!

After Action Report

Any time you're engaging sexually with someone, and especially if you are being game to new experiences, unpacking the experience after the excitement cycle part is over can be incredibly beneficial. Is this something you continue to want on the menu or nah?

Do you feel relaxed? Happy? Calm? Embodied? Satisfied? If this is a person that you have a level of relationship with, do you feel closer to them? These are all signals of a positive experience.

Positivity aside, not everything has to add up to 100 percent amazing. It's also important to ask yourself what you enjoyed specifically...what brough your the most pleasure? What was less pleasurable? What was the most physically intense? Emotionally intense? Did anything surprise you? How so? Was there anything that you struggled to convey in the moment that your partner would have benefits from hearing? Is there anything you wanted to share feedback around?

If you are struggling with some guilt afterward, check in with yourself about whose voice speaks this guilt. If it's external, question that. If whoever speaks with such judgment in your head was silenced (a family member, pastor, society in general) how would you feel? For example, if noone on the planet cared that you liked having sex while wearing an Eeyore onesie, and in fact, were highly encouraging... would you still feel that it was wrong for you? This helps us separate out cultural programming from our own authentic desire.

But...with trauma histories it can be difficult to figure out what is authentic to us, versus the ghosts of past pain. If this is your history, check in with the specifics around that. Did you feel connected or dissociated? Was your entire focus on your partner or did you stop to connect to your own pleasure (because yes, giving is also supposed to be pleasurable)? If you find that you perform well with a partner but struggle with being truly present I'd like to strongly, strongly suggest a therapist who works specifically with trauma because you deserve authentic pleasure, too!

Communication Strategies

Virginia Satir was a therapist and author, often referred to as the mother of family therapy, whose work on resolving communication has been used for decades. She found in her practice as a clinical social worker, that change could be affected fairly quickly by identifying issues with communication and working to improve communication effectiveness.

She theorized that our issues with communication are related to the things we needed to do to survive in our families of origin, which we often carry through to adulthood. This led her to identify patterns in our communication strategies and create a model around them. The first four communication strategies (placating, computing, blaming, distracting) emerge as shields. We aren't being deliberately shitty, we're being trauma reactive and self-protective...even when these strategies no longer serve.

PLACATERS

Placaters agree. They tend to do things to please others, to their own detriment. The body posture and voice often demonstrate subservience to the person they are trying to placate. The internet often refers to this as fawning behavior.

BLAMERS

Blamers always disagree as a show of power and autonomy. They may demonstrate intimidating behavior in the process, such as a loud voice / aggressive stance / threatening behaviors. Blamers are the most likely to initiate conflict, but that drive generally comes from feeling very alienated.

COMPUTERS

Computers are freakily calm and rational even in in heightened emotional conditions. They strive to be ultra-reasonable which can make them seem unmoving around and dismissive of the feelings of others. A computer is ultra-reasonable, rationalizing and trivializing the content of communication.

DISTRACTORS

Distractors don't follow the subject at hand at all. They may seem nonsensical, but they are really working to get away from uncomfortable topics by trying to get everyone to pay attention to something safer. If a topic shift doesn't work, they may ignore questions, drift off, act sleepy, etc.

LEVELER

Levelers are emotionally balanced. They are assertive about their wants and needs without steamrolling others. This doesn't mean they aren't emotional, but it does mean their communication communication is clear regarding their wants and needs and they want problem solving to be beneficial to all parties involved, instead of aiming for some configuration of "you win" or "I win" or "what problem?" Conflict doesn't feel good but it takes less of a toll on their self-worth.

Communication: Noping and Yesing and Feedback Convos

So, clearly the idea is to be a leveler. Satir used the term to describe someone who operates "on the level," meaning with an authenticity and congruence that demonstrates they are trustworthy and engaged. Satir (along with all helping professionals everywhere) demonstrated time and again that we are not our behavior and are entirely capable of recognizing our patterns that no longer serve and adopting new ones.

Leveler communication styles also quickly derail the four more problematic styles quickly because a leveler uses clear language, coming to their point quickly and redirecting back to it when necessary. They ask others to speak for themselves, requests for their feedback, acknowledges their experiences...all without taking on responsibility for anyone but themselves. Levelers address complicated emotions, are responsive to themselves and the people they are talking to, and do not exert pressure on others to follow their will.

Conversations around sex are nerve wracking for most human peoples. After all, this isn't something society encourages us to do. And our extra-annoying narrative around oral sex in particular hasn't helped matters. The only way out of Mordor is through Mordor and the quickest route is to come through with the conscious effort of a badass leveler who goes in wanting to solve the problem, not win an argument.

(When working with couples, I challenge many arguments in my office with "Ok, is this the two of you against the problem or the two of you against each other?")

"No, thank you" to something you don't want to do isn't mean. It's clear. And clear is always the kindest option. If you're struggling with that, I feel ya, and I highly recommend my book *Unfuck Your Boundaries*.

The biggest obstacle to overcome in saying no, and often even to a conditional yes, besides our own internal people pleasing instincts, is to make sure we are differentiating that the no is a rejection of an offer, not a rejection of the other person or your relationship with them. Having a few back-pocket scripts can be hugely beneficial if you struggle to express yourself. Such as:

1) I'm super into you, but that particular activity is not on my menu. It's like shellfish, most people love it and others are allergic.

2) I'm ready to get started. Do you prefer to put on a condom yourself or is it sexier if I help?

3) I can tell you had a long day at work, let's take a shower together and get refreshed before we get into bed.

4) I love how into receiving you are from me, it turns me on. But receiving from you is also a huge turn on and I'd like more of that in our life. Without making it a weird scoring system or something, how can we be more equitable in sexitimes?

THE FEEDBACK BURRITO

Sometimes we realize something isn't great for us, during or after the fact. This is utterly normal and natural and you aren't expected to know everything and express it perfectly. And you are allowed to realize that something you were game to try is not something you want to continue to do. Or that you still like the idea but y'all didn't do great on the execution. One skill I learned in my doc program[8] was how to give feedback to new interns in a way that

8 From Dr. Heather Trepal. I'm saying that for the sole purpose of embarrassing her by mentioning her in a book about cunnilingus with the word fuck in the title.

incorporated all the things they were doing really, really right with the area that we needed to work on. It's slightly more complicated than sandwich feedback (positive, negative, positive), because the human brain centers negative information so strongly (for survival reasons).

This means taking a little extra care in communicating, knowing that brains can be total negativity trolls, by encouraging while also requesting change. Hence the term burrito because the formula is: positive comment, positive comment, place we need to do a little work, positive comment.

Example:

I loved it when you did _____

And _____ was smokin' hot

One thing I think would work better if we did it differently is _____ . I think it would be even better if we _____ instead of _____ next time.

And all in all, I really enjoyed _____.

So, all in all, we are putting the request for something different rolled up with lots of praise.

HOW TO GIVE CUNNILINGUS

Ok, this is the part you showed up for, right?[9] Tips and tricks for tongue stuff. Sometimes it feels a little silly to write introductory paragraphs for the blatantly obvious, so let's just stoodis. Firsties, though? Anatomy lesson.

Anatomy of a Pelvic Area of Someone Born with a Vulva

The pelvic area of the garden variety/no visible indicators of an intersex condition) human is just as complicated and wild to contemplate as that of all the other varieties of humans. We don't think of it that way because more of it seems visible but there is still plenty going on on the inside. For now we are going to mostly focus on the external parts, but as we complete these levels we will move into some internals that may be fun for all involved parties. First of all, there is not that big of a difference between the genitals of people born with a penis and those born with a vagina, check it:

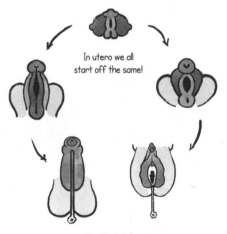

In utero we all start off the same!

How Genitals Develop

---

9 And I want SO MUCH CREDIT for not saying "the part you came for." Except, whoopsie.

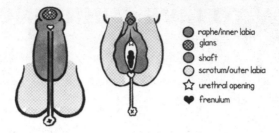

legend:
- raphe/inner labia
- glans
- shaft
- scrotum/outer labia
- ☆ urethral opening
- ♥ frenulum

Ok, now the specific break down of the different parts of the vulva:

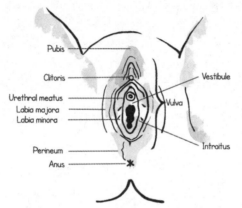

Pubis

Clitoris

Urethral meatus
Labia majora
Labia minora

Perineum
Anus

Vestibule

Vulva

Introitus

And the vagina is actually part of the vulva (not the other way around) and looks like this:

We have a very specific idea of how labia should look, but there is no normal standard on any

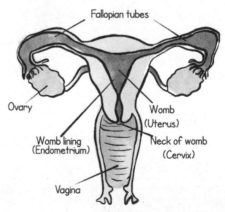

Fallopian tubes

Ovary

Womb lining
(Endometrium)

Vagina

Womb
(Uterus)

Neck of womb
(Cervix)

human lips—the ones on our face or the ones on our labia. Some labia are curved, some are asymmetrical, some have inner lips that hang lower than the labia, among other variations. Tl;dr there is no "normal" other than *your* normal.

Now, the clitoris? Is pretty damn magical:

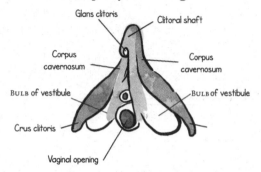

In the neverending theme of not being that invested in the health of people with vulvas, we did not have a clear understanding of how intricate and cool and big the clitoris actually is. Funding research requires pitching that there is some level of problem to be solved. And since the sole function of the clitoris is pleasure . . . and its not the pleasure of cis men…no research funding sources gave one flying fuck.

Way after we knew about the internal structure of penes, we started using MRIs to study the internal structure of the clitoris. In 1998, a urologist named Helen O'Connell from the Royal Melbourne Hospital published her findings on the structure of the nerve supply to the clitoris using this technology, and after continuing her research, published another study in 2005 demonstrating that the clitoris actually extends beyond the vaginal wall.

During this same time period, two doctors named Odile Buisson and Pierre Foldès were working to improve techniques to treat victims of vulva mutilation (generally referred to as female genital mutilation). Once again, no funding was allocated, but they spent their own funds and three years in order to complete the first sonographic map of the erect clitoris (even though the MRI technology to do so has existed for many years). This map was published in 2009.

So first off, I nominate these three doctors to have their faces placed on the modern sainthood candles. Second of all, we learned so much more about the clitoris in the past few years than in all the decades before, combined.

Though I'm not particularly bothered if anyone wants to bring back calling it the devil's teat.

Clitorides range in length from 7 to 12 centimeters, most of which is internal not external. They have more than 8000 nerve endings (twice that of penes) and they swell when engorged, from 50% up to 300%. The swelling increases through excitement to climax. They are made of a mixture of erectile tissue, nerves, and muscles, creating more than 18 distinct parts.

The outside part we most think ourselves fond of is the *glans*. The word glans derives from the Latin word for acorn, which I appreciate. Not to be confused with *glands* which are bodily organs that produce substances, glans as in a highly innervated body of tissue. They exist on the human body as the head of a penis or head of a clitoris. The whole rest of the clitoris is the innie parts.

There are two *corpora cavernosa* (corpus cavernosum for both of them together) which wrap around the vagina from either side like squid tentacles. Then they branch off again forming the two *crura* (crus for both of them together). The crus extends out like two more tentacles, that point down toward the thighs when not erect, and stretch back to the spine when all hot and bothered. These tentacles extend out and attach to the cartilaginous joint known as the symphysis that is part of the pelvic girdle. This particular joint is in front of and below the bladder.

Got all that? Ready for the anatomy quiz? Wait, there's more! Near each crura are the clitoral vestibules, which are on either side of the vaginal opening and under the labia majora. Because all parts of the clitoris get engorged, this is why the vaginal opening feels sensitive and tighter. It's not the cave itself but the cave opening.

Ok, just one more fun fact then I'll move on, I swear. Every part of the human body ages, right? Everything gets saggier, hairier, and spottier except clitorides. It is the only part of the human body that ages not a bit. You can hand over any other part of the body and scientists could age that part. But your clitoris at 97 looks no different than your clitoris at 17. Magical little squid.

Getting Started

So we are gonna start slowly rather than just bury our face in someone's crotch, right? Now of course you aren't going to scream "pull off your pants, it's time for me to go clam diving!" I mean, unless that's y'all's thing. While you're fooling around, you can press your thigh and rub between your partners legs which provides more friction than just using a couple of fingers. Then as you head down south you can get more specific with your fingers and lips, pressing through the fabric of their clothes to tease the clitoral glans.

Once clothing is removed, you can do the discreet check for sores/cuts/scabs and any off-smelling discharge that may signal some kind of bacterial or fungal infection, plus pull out any STI barrier methods y'all's are using (sex dam, gloves, etc).

In order to isolate the clitoris, part the labia. A turned-on clitoris will be the only part that isn't soft when your fingers explore the area. If it seems particularly shy, you can press gently (in and up) on your partner's mons (the fatty tissue area that lies over the vulva and the top of the pelvic structure).

Once you find it, you can use your lips to gently draw it out even more, and your tongue to push back the clitoral hood and get more direct access (unless that's too much stimulation…if they start scooching away from you abort mission). Then run your tongue over the entirety of the glans to get your partner going. If they like extra sensation, you can use your lips to create some light suction.

Generally speaking, we best orgasm through stimulation that is rhythmic and consistent. You don't need to get fancy and draw out the alphabet with your tongue or any of that crap. Pay attention to your partner's cues. Let them adjust in order to increase their comfort, your access, and their sensory experience rather than adjust with them.

If they start grinding toward your mouth, let them control the movement and speed by leaving your tongue flat (or curled if you are able to do that) under their clitoris while they ride against it. But if they go completely still, that's also a good sign to keep doing exactly what you are doing exactly how you are doing it until they orgasm.

Make noises of enjoyment, especially if your partner is strongly auditory. Slurping noises and hums of satisfaction will be a turn on to them (and the humming can produce some vibratory sensations that they also enjoy. Remember as you speed up that you want to create and maintain a solid rhythm for your partner. You don't want to go so fast as vinyl on an RPM setting that makes everything sound like Alvin and The Chipmunks, right?

Breathing feeling difficult? Slow back down (and obviously stop ANYTHING you are uncomfortable with), try the breathing techniques suggested in the next section, try pulling back a little and letting only the tip of your tongue and/or your fingers do most of the work. Some people find that the gag reflex sprays (that add a little numbing to your mouth and throat) can also be helpful.

But what if they start pushing down on your head? First off, rude. Definitely an after-action report issue to discuss. But in the moment if you don't want to disrupt proceedings, lightly grab their hand or wrist, remove it off your head and set it back down on the bed or their lap and say "I got this, just relax and let me do the work" and keep going.

BREATHE FOR HEAD

Generally speaking your face lips are going to be horizontal while their vulva lips are going to be vertical, so if you breathe through your mouth you should be fine. If you are struggling with tongue action and mouth breathing at the same time and need to use your nose, you can shift your body perpendicular to theirs, which also allows you to place a pillow under your head for support.

For those of you who thought that playing woodwind at band camp would never make you sexy? My two words for you are *circular breathing*. Now y'all already have it down, but it is an easy skill for the rest of us to learn as it's just a breathing technique that allows you to switch back and forth between breathing through your lungs and cheeks. You can find a lot of instructions and demo videos online and you can practice the technique using a straw and a glass of water until you get it down.

TEMPERATURE AND SENSORY PLAY

The possibilities are nigh endless here, aren't they? This is where you can get super creative fairly inexpensively. For temperature play you can incorporate ice, something cold and bubbly (La Croix or whatever floats your boat since it's going in your mouth), or something warm and soothing (hot tea is great...mint tea will add a little bit of a tingle). You can alternate between hot and cold as well. Unlike with penes, you want to avoid using anything that has sugar content (like pop rocks, champagne, sugar soda, etc).[10] Sugar *down there* is a gnarly infection waiting to happen.

You can also use touch based sensory items over their body, like silk scarves, while you work the glans with your tongue.

SEX TOYS! ERM, I MEAN TOOLS. SEX TOOLS!

A lot of people have a sense of unease about incorporating sex aids into their partnered or unpartnered sexual activity. Societal messages (religious or otherwise) often attach a sense of shame to the use of sexual aids, even if sexual intimacy itself is not judged.

---

10 I did look. There are popping candies marketed specifically for oral sex but all of them have sugar. Until a keto version is created, don't put them in your mouth before burying your mouth onto a vulva.

But there are many reasons that using sexual aids may be exactly the right thing for you and/or your relationship.

Sexual aids can:

- Be a lifesaver if you're experiencing physical limitations to your sexual expression. For example, individuals who struggle to maintain an erection might find that a hollow core strap allows them to have penetrative intercourse with their partner. Or people with limited mobility can use remote control operated vibrators to masturbate to orgasm, which is incredibly empowering if you have had to rely on others for that experience in the past.

- Be used in a partnership to facilitate increased intimacy and overcome performance limitations with either partner.

- Provide an experience within partnerships that is otherwise out of the comfort zone of one of the partners (such as anal stimulation or BDSM activities).

- Allow people to be authentically who they are. A traditional strap-on can allow someone to participate in penetrative intercourse if they don't have a penis, for instance. Other companies have started producing FTM specific stroker toys, designed specifically to allow transmen the stroking sensation that other men enjoy, while taking into account that they have larger genitalia due to gender confirmation hormone treatment.

- Provide extra stimulation. Some people just need more stimulation to orgasm and aids can provide that without exhausting either partner or having them develop anxiety about trying to please their partners.

- Facilitate intimacy in long distance relationships. There are devices designed to provide pleasure to a partner from afar, such as Bluetooth-controlled vibrators...the best thing for long distance relationships since Skype sex!

- And sexual aids are just fun! I've had many people tell me that they were not in need of any assistance, but when they tried something new (such as a lubricant), they say, "Wow, okay, so much better!"

Probably the biggest question folks have is "will I break my junk?" Meaning, if they use something that provides a LOT of stimulation will it ruin me for what a partner does. Short answer? No. While some people do better with extra stimulation (and you may therefore use things with a partner), you won't stop feeling your partner's touch. If anything, think of it as taking a walk or taking a train. Both have benefits. You can slow down and enjoy the scenery and your own motion getting you somewhere, or you can be less scenic about your journey in order to save time. You get there either way.

We've already talked about using a fizzy drinks, tea and other such shenanigans. Guess what? Those are also sex tools. They're enhancements you show up to the party with, just like it's a bottle of Cinco and a quart of juice. Except this is edible lube for extra slurpies or whatever.

Sex tools are getting more non-gender specific as society remembers that humans have never ascribed to an immutable binary. Tools like the PicoBong Transformer, which is a sister brand of Lelo, can be used as a massager, a rabbit, an erection ring, a double ended vibrator or a double ended dildo. Like a utility tool for all your household needs.

So consider this big permission to experiment with anything that may help you have more satisfying adventures.

THE G SPOT

We discussed in detail some of the historical fuckery around sexual pleasure in general and oral sex specifically. Freud wasn't opposed so much to those things in general, but was still quite certain that if a woman was psychologically mature, she could have vaginal orgasms. If a woman continued to focus on clitoral pleasure she would develop a mental health disorder soon after. Then not long later, in 1950, the G spot was discovered, though that wasn't what it was called until German gynecologist Ernst Gräfenberg[11] referred to "an erotic zone always could be demonstrated on the anterior wall of the vagina along the course of the urethra" when studying the role of urethra stimulation in the orgasms of someone with a vulva.

He piggybacked on what Dutch physician Regnier de Graaf noted in the 17th century regarding female ejaculation in what he called an erogenous zone in the vagina that he thought operated similarly to the male prostate. The name Gräfenberg spot, or G spot, actually came from a team of researchers led by Frank

---

11 Dr. Gräfenberg was hella interesting and needs his own biopic made STAT. He was the head of the OB/GYN branch of a hospital in Germany and stepped down from that role when the Nazis took power, but didn't leave. He thought that although he was Jewish he treated the wives of many high ranking Nazi party officials. He was wrong. They didn't kill him but held him in a Nazi prison for several years until Margaret Sanger paid the ransom for his release and he was able to move to New York to continue his work studying the female orgasm and inventing a better IUD.

Addiego who were also studying female ejaculation and gave old Ernst the credit for the find.

What area are they referring to? An area up in the front part of the vaginal wall about 2-3 inches (5-8 cm) inward. Stimulating that area with a penis, fingers, or toy can lead to strong orgasms and female ejaculation.

But! As we now know! Only since 2009 but still! The vaginal cavity isn't actually that sensitive in and of itself, and now that we have properly mapped an aroused clitoris the area being stimulated is actually the internal part of the clitoris. The root of the corpus cavernosum specifically.

It's still a clitorial orgasm, so suck it Freud.

Also, it's important to say that if that stimulation doesn't do anything for you, you aren't doing anything wrong. Since the G spot is actually a mythical beast in and of itself, stimulation of the corpus cavernosum may not connect in your body to some

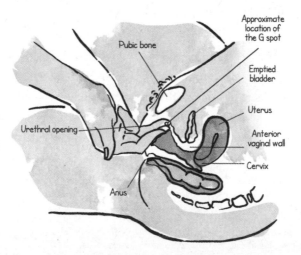

mythical vaginal wall place. It may be elsewhere on the top of your vaginal wall or not at all. So if you are hitting this area on a partner and it isn't doing anything for them? You aren't doing things wrong, everyone has natural body variations, just go back to focusing on their glans.

PERIOD CUNNILINGUS

Ok, what are menses exactly? I never learned the specifics in school, maybe you didn't either. There are epithelial cells (which are cells that just line surfaces throughout your body…like your skin) that line the uterus along with strong connective tissue and lots of blood vessels. This lining is created by the body monthly in case an egg gets fertilized with the potential to grow into a fetus. If that doesn't happen, the body activates a hormone shift that tells the uterus to dump the nest it built. All these cells and connective tissue shed and blood vessels break in the process. So that's why we see blood. And that stuff that looks like clots is usually that actual lining.

There is less actual blood than it looks and feels like. Even though those of us who menstruate may feel like *Carrie* at the prom[12], it's really only about two shot glasses of blood over several days. So during sexual activity, espeically if you are supine, you may not see any blood unless you are in the middle of that Day 2 heavy rush. If you notice that the blood seems really bright, like you would expect from a wound, that is quite likely not period blood and they do have some kind of injury they need to know about and get treated.

---

12 Look up this scene from the movie *Carrie*, adapted from the Stephen King novel of the same name if you don't get the reference or want a visual refresher.

The health risks associated with having sex with a menstruating partner are super lower. There is a slightly higher risk of transmitting a blood-borne STI (like syphilis and HIV), which is easily managed with the barrier methods described later in this book.

Or, if you aren't into the blood, you can again use a barrier method. Additionally your partner can use a tampon or a menstrual cup or disk[13] to capture the flow before it exits the vaginal canal. You can also use a towel (suggest a darker one) or a puppy training pad (disposable) to capture any leakage. Depending on the fabric, hydrogen peroxide is also really good at getting out blood if you spill a bit.

Because there is also increased blood flow and reduced estrogen to that entire region, not just *exiting that* entire region, it can actually be great for orgasming. If your partner has uncomfortable period symptoms (cramps, bloating, all that fun stuff) then an orgasm can actually help alleviate a lot of those symptoms[14] and oral sex tends to be more comfortable than penetrative sex when their body is already cranky about the state of affairs.

If your partner gets pelvic floor pain, they may be more comfortable having some support under their lower back or pulling their legs up while lying on their back. My yogi peeps can attest that if you can do so comfortably, the reclining bound angle

13 If you are doing any clitoral stimulation from inside the vaginal canal (you know, fingering) be aware that a tampon will absorb not just menses but vaginal lubrication so it might not be a pleasant sensation as it is for the rest of the month. Because the other menstruation products sit higher, they don't absorb the body's natural lubrication and may be more comfortable. Also? Lube will forevermore be your friend if needed…if you don't make your own store bought is fine!

14 Clinical research published in 2020 found that 42% of menstruating individuals found symptom relief from masturbation. The study was funded by a sex toy company. Zero shame in that, but that led to headlines that didn't point out it was the *orgasm* that was helpful. Self-induced is great but so is partner induced.

form (Supta Baddha Konasana) or one of its variations can be very helpful and good for partner access.

A lot of people are uncomfortable with partnered activity when they are on their period, as if it is something shameful versus a regular part of life. Don't push them if they don't want to, but you can also remind them that you wouldn't do something you're not down for and have no problem with their body. And some people are super into period cunnilingus. Blood hounds dig the musky smell and more metallic taste of their partner's body during that time period. Because this is what happens if you are my neighbor....I did bug my friend/neighbor who is a biker about earning a red wings patch. He says it's not a thing really anymore but it was back in the day, thanks Lance!

THE VARIETIES OF WAP

Not all fluids released during sex are the same thing, especially if you have a vulva. The term vaginal discharge is usually thought of as some sign of infection, but it really relates to any fluid that comes out of the vagina. For example, it's entirely normal to discharge up to a teaspoon of mucus-like discharge daily. As long as it is white or clear and is odorless it's totally fine. It's mucus, water, and shedding cells, nbd. The signs that there may be a health issue like a bacterial infection, yeast infection, or trichomoniasis (which is an STI) are:

- Color changes (greenish, yellowish, brownish that isn't menses)

- Increase in volume along with other symptoms like itching

- Texture changes (gets way thinner or thicker)

- Smell (fishy, metallic, generally not pleasant)

Because hormones fluctuate throughout the month for individuals that are ovulating, menstruating, or pregnant your partner may notice that they are wetter closer to ovulation and drier during menses because of those estrogen changes. This is less the case if you are on a hormonal birth control or your body no longer cycles in this way due to surgery, menopause, etc.

When we talk about "getting wet" we are talking about the cervical fluid that the body releases for penetrative intercourse. It's caused by the increased genital blood flow which creates pressure for transudate fluid to push up to the surface of the vaginal walls. Besides hormonal changes (including birth control or hormone therapy), other medications can affect this process, as can mental health issues, general stress, and lack of foreplay.

It's also super important to remember what we discussed earlier in the book, which is that physical and psychological arousal are not the same thing. Lack of wetness doesn't necessarily mean not interested, and wetness doesn't necessarily mean interested. It's still alllllll about partner communication.

Ok, cool. There is also a difference between vulva ejaculate and squirting from the urethra. If you have seen big fluid releases from a partner or in erotic performance videos and the like it was probably squirting. The fluid released in squirting is at best guess (once again no surprise that we don't really know for sure) is a mix of water, some urine, and maybe a little ejaculate. You will see some articles that say "meh, it's all just urine" which could freak out anyone (unless golden showers are your thing) but as of me writing this, that doesn't seem to be the case. One study looked at not just what was emitted but what was going on with the bladder before and after squirting and it looks like even someone with an empty bladder before sexitimes had a bladder that filled up quickly during sexitimes and squirted *that* fluid. So this speaks to the probability that the body is drawing fluid up for release the way the vaginal walls do.

If it still concerns you, no biggie. Use a barrier method like a sex dam and focus your attention on the clitoral glans which is above the urethra if you are concerned about accidental ingesting.

But wait, there *is* more! Along with wetness and squirting, there is also vulva ejaculate. This fluid isn't clear, but more resembles a diluted milk (as described in the aforementioned witch trial manuscripts . . . so at least that part was accurate). A study in 2013 measured the amount of ejaculate from over 300 participants and found a huge range in volume. From .3 mL to 150mL and more. Which is .06 of a teaspoon to more than half a cup. So no one is ejaculating too much or too little…once again bodies are all interesting and different.

Where does all this fluid come from? Quite likely the Skene's glands. While the Skene's glands were first detailed in the late 1800s by gynecologist Alexander Skene (hence the name), researchers realizing the similarities between these glands and the prostate is really new.

A 2011 study recognized that many of the components of the Skene's gland ejaculate are the same as in semen. Meaning prostate enzymes including prostate specific antigen (PSA) and prostatic acid phosphatase. There are also small amounts of urea and creatine (components of urine) even though the ejaculate is clearly known to not be urine, even among cranky competing scientists.

The glands rest on the front wall of the vagina, and surround the urethra and include openings that allow them to release this ejaculate (it doesn't come from a water filled bladder like squirting does). Researchers published a study in 2017, demonstrating that the glands probably have even more openings than we thought. Or, more specifically, they have the capacity to increase the number of openings they have which is why some individuals ejaculate larger amounts of fluid.

Ok, so I spent a lot of time discussing all the vaginal secretions that are not urine. But are there times it could be urine? Absolutely. Some people do experience urinary incontinence with penetration and orgasm and not otherwise. Kegel exercises can help with this, as can pelvic floor training with a physical therapist and medications. If it really looks and smells like pee, it could be and definitely merits getting checked out.

Can I be….allergic?

Being allergic to semen is rare though not as rare as you would think, either allergic to the seminal plasma itself or an allergy to a food or medication that your partner had taken. This means that it is also possible to be allergic to vaginal secretions though good luck finding info about that online. There are very few mentions of vaginal fluids causing the same reaction. Maybe because vulvae aren't studied as much as penes, but also equally likely that these varieties of vaginal secretions are rarely ingested or deposited.

Besides using barrier methods for protection, allergists do recommend doing an allergy patch test where the particular possible allergen is put on a patch and attached to one's skin to check for a skin inflammation. Since this can all be done at home and is needle free, this would be the most inexpensive and least violating way to test if this is the case.

Cunnilingus Adapted to Disability

The Centers for Disease Control defines disability as "any condition of the body or mind (impairment) that makes it more difficult for the person with the condition to do certain activities (activity limitation) and interact with the world around them (participation restrictions)." So this can include a lot of the different ways we show up in the world. How our brains work (including how they relate to and understand other people and relationships) and how our bodies work. And manymanymany (most) of these disabilities are invisible, or mostly invisible.

Which leads back to (drumrolls and eyerolls please)...having discussions with our partners. The pre-game discussions and the after action reports.

This is another area where sex tools can be incredibly helpful, not just for stimulation but for access. Like a good wedge pillow to help us keep our bodies well supported.

It is also helpful to get creative about positions and communication strategies. Sitting down may be easier for access than lying down, whether you are a giver or a receiver. If you use a chair for mobility, there is not a thing wrong with staying in your chair for support.

If you have pain issues, especially if it gets stabby and spasmy, consider that when you are considering positions. Orgasms can increase those sensations along with the pleasurable ones. So if you are fine now but leg cramping happens on the regular, planning to support your legs juuuuuust in case will make it less likely that it ends up being a complete mood killer.

If mobility/dexterity can be an issue, don't hesitate to ask your partner for assistance. It's ok to ask them to position their genitals to your mouth, for example. You can also give good head while letting a (trusted!) partner do all of the movement stuff, especially helpful if you have neck mobility issues. You can supply the tongue and let your partner control the movement of their hips and pelvis.

Cunnilingus After Vaginoplasty

Vaginoplasty is a procedure to construct or repair a vagina, a labiaplasty is a procedure which focuses specifically on decreasing the size of the labia, and a vulvoplasty is a procedure used to reshape the outer part of the vagina. While all of these procedures include surgical downtime, the vaginoplasty is the one that can have specific follow-up care and considerations for sexitimes later.

Vaginoplasty is used not just as a gender affirming surgical intervention for trans women and transfemme individuals, it is also used to treat a number of medical issues experienced by cis women, including vaginal injury, congenital differences that are posing issues to bodily processes and sexual pleasure, and complications that can arise from pelvic floor disease.

While possible side effects and considerations exist for any of the medically necessary reasons for getting a vaginoplasty, there will be more complications for someone who is getting a fully constructed vagina and vulva than repairing an existing one, such as fistula and stenosis. Most everyone will have some significant healing downtime and may need to continue to use a vaginal dilator to maintain a healthy vaginal canal.

Depending on the surgery (and all those other varieties of human response times), it can take up to a year to recover sensation in that area. And it may take several years for the brain to create new maps about these sensations coming from a different place than before (once again back to the brain being the most important sex organ).

Research is scarce (shocking, I know!) but what is out there shows that trans women have not just the increased blood flow (vasocongestion) but also fluid secretion during sex, and "moderate to high" rates of orgasm functioning post vagioplasty recovery.

The general recommended best practice is for the individual who received the procedure to self-test their sensory responses. This doesn't just mean engaging in solo sex in order to figure out what they like and don't like now (though definitely do that!), but also self testing for sensitivity to pressure, vibration, and temperature changes. Some changes in sensation will hopefully not be permanent. For example, the healing nerves can create some incredible electrical zapping sensations as they reconnect. The good news is the self-testing can help speed up the healing process, because it encourages the brain's sensory map-making.

Studying orgasm and erotic sensations is so complex, individual, and systems-based that it's really hard to study well. The research that is out there shows that individuals who were able to orgasm before vaginoplasty are generally still able to do so, although many report some loss of sensation. Additionally, individuals who were not able to orgasm in the past because of dysphoric distress find they are able to after surgery and their healing period.

Cunnilingus on a No-Op Trans/GNC Partner with a Vulva

The prevailing "wisdom" (read: presumption) is that hormone therapy as a gender confirmation treatment is disruptive to sex drive. And turns out? Not true. Trans women have the same rates of hyposexual desire disorder as those of the general cis-chica population and studies also show that gender confirmation treatment is generally really good for people's sexual expression because you feel better/more authentic/more comfortable in your body when you are your real self.

Knowing that the glans of the penis and the clitoris have the same point of origin in utero (see earlier in this book) can be helpful for a trans man or transmasc individual who enjoys oral stimulation but is also experiencing dysphoria. And once an individual has been on T for awhile, bottom growth may help that process.

Bottom growth is the super non-technical term for the changes that happen to the glans with testosterone therapy. Meaning it grows a little longer (generally not more than 2 inches) and a little thicker (I have found zero research with averages in that regard), depending on dosage and time spent on T.

The growth can feel extra sensitive to the point of discomfort during the first six months of treatment, which may make direct stimulation painful. Hell, even boxer-briefs may rub one the wrong

Ex. pre-testosterone

Ex. unaroused
and/or low dose

Ex. aroused
and/ or high dose

way at that point. Don't take it personally if your partner is not super into sexitimes during this time in their lives.

If you want the other masculinizing effects without bottom growth, or if it's super uncomfortable, a doctor can prescribe a DHT blocker though it will have other side effects (including possibly restarting menses which may have stopped as a result of the hormone treatment).

Is there really much difference in oral sex technique, Nope. We already have so many differences in how and where we like to be touched, and as a good partner you are already asking those questions so you're good to go. The one thing you and your partner may be interested in including are some transmasc specific sex tools.

As you can see that while everyone's miles may vary, the glans may be big enough to use stroking toys and the like as part of sexitimes and some individuals have found that a pump specific for testosterone treated glans does help with their growth and/or appearance as does DHT (the sex hormone dihydrotestosterone), which is a specific compound pharmaceutical that is used specifically on the glans to promote growth. However, cis men who got a phalloplasty to correct a birth defect or injury (versus a non-cis man who had his penis created completely from another area of skin) may get some assistance from these activities, and it's worth asking during surgical follow-up when discussing being released to sexual practice.

Cunnilingus on a No-Op Trans/GNC Partner with a Penis

This is another place where knowing that all glans are essentially the same comes in handy. And plenty of trans women and transfemme peeps still enjoy oral pleasure. There are also several specific techniques if you are going for expert level eating out. I highly recommend *Girl Sex 101* by Allison Moon, specifically the section that she titles "Girl Dick Bean Lick" where she describes techniques including the genital bouquet (which involves using your hands to bundle together your partner's genital area so you can work your tongue around the whole area easily) and the flying squirrel (which involves pulling the scrotum up over the top of the glans before oral stimulation). These techniques can feel great for a non-cis partner since they focus on scrotal stimulation, which is what is the labia on someone born with a vagina, and what becomes the labia if one ends up having vagioplasty. Another great book with not just oral sex techniques but other fun things to experiment with, including muffing (penetration of the inguinal canal with a partner's finger or one's own testical), is Mira Belleweather's book *FTW (Fucking Trans Women)*.

Cunnilingus with an Intersex Partner

It is actually really difficult to identify the difference between intersex and perisex people. We all have stronger and weaker expressions of the different characteristics we term male and female. That being said, the prevailing statistic is 2%. 2% of people have hormones, chromosomes, and/or physical anatomy that varies from our traditional understanding of biological sex. Which also means most intersex people are not going to present with visible anatomical differences to a partner, but they may have different concentrations of hormones affecting their desire rates, their sensitivity, their ability to achieve and maintain erectile tissue, etc.

If your partner has visible anatomical differences, the most important thing for you to know is that you're still going to be focusing on erectile tissue in one place. Remember all that stuff about the penis and clitoris developing from the same organ system? The term for that is homologs, so you can have one or the other or something in between but not both a penis and a clitoris. So when you see news stories about someone who is intersex having both male and female sexual organs? Clearly not just wrong but biologically impossible.

When we are talking about visible differences, and characteristics of both sexes, we are talking about a body that looks like one of the following:

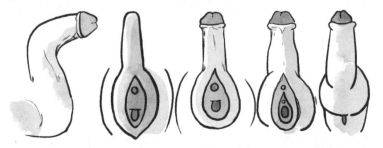

And just like this book is not intended to be a "choose your own surgical adventure," it's also not meant to be an Intersex 101 guide. But it is a fellatio guide! And since bodies come in many variations it's important to honor that and think about how we share sexual pleasure with partners of our bodies right? So we want to discuss with a partner where and how we want to be touched. Where are our sensitive areas? What feels good and what feels less good? And these questions remain true for all bodies, not just for partners with a natural body variation. And if they do have a natural variation there may be other information to consider. For example, are they interested in any penetration of their vaginal canal? They may not have a fully developed vaginal canal, more of a pouch in that area (vaginal agenesis) which could lead to sensations that are uncomfortable or even painful. Also knowing their surgical history will be important. Many individuals with visible variations are operated on when they are very young without their consent by panicked doctors and family members. They may have scar tissue to contend with and/or medical trauma surrounding that area of their body that you will want to be aware and respectful of.

And just like with any other partner, you will want to have discussions about disease transmission, and yes we are going to discuss getting clever with STI protection and different body types later in this book!

HOW TO RECEIVE CUNNILINGUS

Being a polite receiver is about consideration and communication. What can you do to be a considerate receiver right off the bat and how do you figure out the rest? There are definitely some thou shalt nots to keep in mind, though all thou-shalt and thou-shalt-nots are also *situationally dependent*. Maybe your vibe with your partner includes a little kink play that involves something that would otherwise be a default no. Have fun in that space as long as everyone knows what the scene includes.

- Thou shalt not ignore thyne hygiene. Presume that a day at work and a sweaty bike ride home did a number on your concha and your naglas. Even if you don't smell it, someone's face down there definitely will. Err on the side of caution and fresh up for sexitimes.

- Thou shalt consider some trimming as well. Pubic hair protects sensitive skin (and also serves as increasing surface area of your body for releasing pheromones). But a lot of pubic hair can get in the way of partnered shenanigans. Getting yourself some inexpensive clippers and using a guard on them so you don't buzz yourself itchy bald is generally considered good manners. Your hashi will also be more easily accessible to your partner that way.

- Thou shalt not shove someone's head down onto you. Enough said?

- Thou shalt have a plan for fluids. A towel? A puppy training pad?

- Thou shalt discuss if your receiving is supposed to be a warm up for other activities or if you are meant to return the favor. Being able to languish in enjoyment is totally fine as long as your partner is good with giving without expectation of immediate return.

- Thou shalt make eye contact, be complimentary and gracious and grateful. And anything that didn't go well is discussed carefully and possibly with a feedback burrito.

- There haven't been any studies regarding possible connection between diet and the flavor and scent of vaginal discharges, but lots of people have reported that eating sweeter foods does increase the sweetness of these fluids.

Emotional and Medical Concerns

Earlier in the book we talked about how things can change due to different circumstances and times in our lives. Whether for the better or for the more frustrating, different means making adjustments. This part of the book is designed to be as granular as possible around a lot of these options.

Adapting to Your Body

While a lot of this chapter is about adapting our bodies, I want to start with slowing down and caring for our bodies first. It may not change anything about how your body sexually responds, but it will definately change your relationship with that response. And time spent on caring for your body and your health in general is never wasted, trust the clinician nutritionist.

Where Does Desire Come From?

Whenever I am working with anyone on their issues surrounding intimacy, I start by reminding them that sexual desire is something that is within us that we then choose to share with a partner. Sexual desire isn't something somebody else gives us. Even if they are smokin' hot (Paul Rudd, call me!).

One of the first things we do is figure out what helps them feel most in tune to their own sexual selves. Do they feel better when they have time to work out, when they eat a certain way, when they get a day to themselves to rest and not answer emails? This self-care based on self-knowledge work is foundational to everything else.

So let's start there:

• When in your life did you feel best in your body?

• What supported that experience for you?

• What would help you reclaim that in the present?

• What can you start doing this week?

Pleasure Mapping

Sex educator Kenneth Play uses the term *pleasure mapping* to describe the process of connecting to how you enjoy the sensations of your body. This is another level in from connecting to your innate sexual desire, plus creates space for creating and intensifying new erotic pathways.

Because one of the coolest things about having a human body is how ready the brain is at creating new sexual stimulation pathways. We think of pleasure and orgasm as depending on the stimulation of our genitals and research continues to show that's clearly untrue.

Brains are creating new neural pathways all the time, and remapping your senses in order to achieve sexual satisfaction through other parts of the body and in other ways. And if I was reading this right now, I would be thinking "ok, so how the fuck do we do that?" so I imagine you are, too. While my book *Unfuck Your Intimacy* goes into detail about sensate focus exercises, this is actually really different. Where sensate focus is about connecting to the joy of touching your partner's body, pleasure mapping is about connecting to the joy of being touched by others.

Try slowing way down with your partner and pay attention to how and where your body responds:

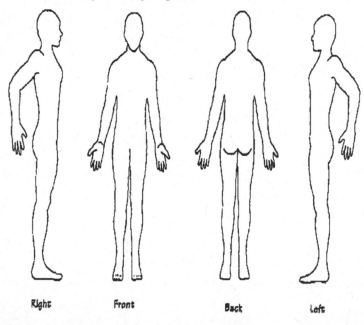

Right   Front   Back   Left

- What kind of pressure do you enjoy?

- How intense?

- What kind of rhythm and movement?

- What positions are you most comfortable in? What about what position your partner is in?

- Is there anything else you noticed?

Stress Management

While we all know a few stress divas who seem to have a homing beacon for inviting stress in, most of us don't choose stress, we just have to deal with it. Stress is our sense of overwhelm or struggle to cope with the mental/emotional aspects of pressure in our lives. Whether it's everyday stress, life events stress, or disintegration of society stress, this is the shitshow we've been handed. And research shows the more we try to avoid stress, the worse it gets. So what does help?

There's good news, I swear there is good news. Research supports that we have far more control over our experience of stress and how it affects our bodies than you'd think. Not by chucking everything and living in a van down by the river, but by changing your perception of stress.

Some smart people compared the National Health Interview Survey data to mortality data in the US. They found that stress alone isn't so bad for you.

Embracing Stress Through Mindset Training

The author of the book *The Upside of Stress*, Kelly McGonigal, (whose research is the starting point for a lot of what I write about here) states: "Embracing stress is a radical act of self trust."

We've been told not to though, haven't we? We're told to avoid stress, to calm down, that it isn't good for us. Harvard Business School professor Alison Wood Brooks asked hundreds of people the same question: If you are anxious about a big presentation, what's a better way of handling it? Feeling excited or trying to calm down?

91% of people said "try to calm down."

But the stress isn't in and of itself bad—it's not necessarily a problem you need to solve or get away from. This is borne out by multiple studies, including the one mentioned above, where the researchers found that just saying "I'm excited" out loud can reappraise stress as excitement. Despite what most of us have been told, it's easier for the brain to jump from anxious feelings to excited ones rather than calm ones. Cortisol is going to be activated because something matters to you. But you can consciously label it as excited instead of stressed, which changes how you interpret and experience your own body.

The practice of reframing our thoughts from those of overwhelm to those of empowerment is known as mindset training. Mindsets are really nothing more than the beliefs we have about ourselves and the world that shape our realities. This isn't negating the fact that we may be dealing with really fucked up situations, but is about taking back whatever power we have in our own responses when dealing with shitshow scenerios.

One of the biggest predictors of stress overwhelming us is our perception of not being up to the task, so focusing on the fact that we are, indeed, up to it shifts our thinking.

It's super important that you don't beat yourself up for not doing stress well. The entire engine of modern society operates on the psychic energy of people not doing stress well. The whole game is designed to work that way. If you are exhausted, burned out, depleted, experiencing adrenal fatigue, and the like, just changing your mindset isn't going to resolve all that.

It took years if not decades to get you to the point of exhaustion you are sitting at right now, right? You can't unfuck this level of attack on a human body by chanting "I'm not stressed, I'm excited!"

Any stressful situation can become an opportunity to practice a mindset shift. When you notice your stress response activating, you can remind yourself that your body is reacting to something because it's important to you. Then, use that energy to help carry you through the situation. Whether you are getting through a stressful interview or fighting facism, being alert, engaged, and present is vital to success.

Mindset training seems awkward at first, but once you build that neural pathway it becomes more natural and more likely to be your automatic response. As you practice, you won't have to work so hard at it over time. Your stress mindset will also change how you react to others' stress. Mindset leads to resilience. And emotional resilience is one of the first lines of defense against mental illnesses like depression and learning what behaviors build that up could clue physicians in on how to treat those illnesses.

Having a GOOD Mindset

You can practice mindset training as part of your daily self-care routine. I like the GOOD acronym of mindset training since it doesn't involve any kind of fake hype about shitty situations, it really just is about being grounded in your own self-efficacy. And clearly you are a fucking survivor—you're reading this right now, which means your survival rate thus far is 100%, right? This is one of those internal work exercises that might be easier to make external by journaling through it, especially at first while you get used to the process. But I am, for once, not insisting you write everything down if you really hate that shit!

Gratitude: Focusing on gratitude is a really good part of our mental health in general and can create a perspective shift in our day. This doesn't mean discounting what's problematic, but focusing more on what's good in your life.

Openness to Possibilities: If we are gratitude focused, we are far more likely to be aware of solutions, support, and opportunities around us. In a negative mindset, we are more likely to dismiss things that are available to us (or not notice them at all) because we are overwhelmed and frustrated with life in general.

Opportunities in this Experience: No matter what experience we are having, we can focus on the opportunities that exist to help us grow. We can learn more about different situations and ourselves even if we don't achieve the success we were hoping for. As someone who does a lot of political advocacy work, I can tell you that every lost battle taught me a new strategy of approach for next time.

Determine: Visualize yourself successfully embracing the challenges ahead. This is hardiness in action. If you mentally set yourself up for success, you are in the right frame of mind to tackle the project. And no, you aren't more frustrated if things don't go perfectly. I've found that even when I don't succeed, I'm still proud of myself for going in prepared and positive because I feel like I really gave it my all.

NUTRITION AND ENVIRONMENT

While there is no magical dietary formula to assist with sexual desire and orgasm capability, I've worked with a lot of people who have created significant improvement in that area by decreasing their processed food intake, adding whole food supplements and/or quality herbs, and even experimenting with their bodies' responses to electromagnetic fields.

I know this all sounds super suspicious, like I am now going to try to sell you on some weird product package that costs thousands of dollars. Actually the opposite is true. Small dietary changes can have a huge effect and (apart from the fact that better quality food costs more) it's free to try. Turning off wireless in your house and/or putting your phone in airplane mode while you sleep? Free to try. And you don't need wifi access when your conked out anyway.

Good quality supplements can be (ok, are) more expensive but can also be incredibly helpful. Typically I look at supplements that support the body's sex hormones (tribulus, ginseng, selinium) and response to stress (adaptogenic herbs like rhodioloa, ashwaganda and the like).

If this route is more your speed, it really is of benefit to consult with a nutritionist who works in this area for an individualized plan. So often people say "just give me a meal plan and tell me what to take" and there are so many more personal factors at play. I like looking at individual symptoms and lab work if it's available. Sometimes there is something going on like a zinc deficiency that is having a cascade effect throughout the body and is easily corrected.

KEGELS

Being healthy is far easier if we exercise, right? Sexual health has its own exercise...the kegel. Obviously, kegels aren't magically curative for all kinds of sexual disorders but they are one of the go-to exercises that really help a lot of people! Kegel exercises are designed to strengthen the pelvic floor muscles, focusing specifically on the "PC" (pubococcygeus) muscles. Kegels have tons of practical use for all kinds of issues, whether you have a vagina or penis.

Dr. Arnold Kegel was a gynecologist who developed these exercises for people who had pelvic floor weakening post-childbirth. He found another interesting side benefit: His patients who were doing kegels regularly were achieving orgasm with greater ease and frequency, and had a more intense experience, showing that kegels have an additional benefit to sexual intimacy. They have been found to help both women and men better achieve orgasm, and can help both sexes feel more in control of their sexual experience for a few reasons:

- Kegels help control urinary incontinence, so many individuals feel more secure during sexual activity and less likely to leak urine.

- Kegels help give the individual on the receiving end of penetrative intercourse more control over the experience and more intense orgasms. They also create a tighter vagina or anus, therefore increasing the pleasure of the penetrating partner as well.

- Kegels help bring more blood flow to the pelvic region in women and the perineum region in men, potentially intensifying your arousal.

Kegels can be done with or without an aid (such as a dildo, vibrator, or tool designed specifically for kegel mastery like Betty Dodson's kegelcizer). They can be done solo (which is usually a good place to start) as well as during penetrative intercourse (which can be a lot of fun for both partners).

Here's how to do them:

- Locate the muscle group in question by squeezing the muscles you use to stop your urine flow. If you are urinating and are able to halt the flow, you have the right muscle group. Your stomach and buttocks muscles should not tighten in the process. You also don't want to do your kegel exercises when emptying your bladder on a regular basis. That can lead to weakening the pelvic floor muscles which can prevent you from fully emptying your bladder (which, in turn, can lead to an increase in urinary tract infections).

- If you are using a kegel aid, lubricate the aid before insertion and practice kegels lying down. If you are not using an aid, it may be of benefit at first to practice lying down.

- Squeeze the muscle group for three seconds, then release for three seconds. Complete 10 to 15 cycles of squeeze and release.

- Try to do this at least three times a day. The more regularly you perform the exercise, the better results you will get (just like any exercise).

As you get more comfortable doing this, you will find that you don't have to set aside "kegel time" to be effective. You can do them while engaging in other activities since no one will know what you are up to—unless of course you are doing them during sex, in which case your partner will know and appreciate it.

MEDICATIONS, CREAMS, AND SHOTS OH MY

Depending on your symptoms and the other stuff you and your prescriber notice that is going on, many people end up getting good benefit from hormone therapy, which can be administered as a pill, cream, or vaginal suppository. Several hormone treatments have been associated with a restoration of sexual functioning, including estrogen, estrogen receptor modulators, testosterone, androgens, and steroids such as tibolone, Other commonly used off label treatments include bupropion (Wellbutrin/Zyban) which has a positive libido effect and erectile dysfunction medications like Viagra (cuz glans is glans is glans).

Now the only two medications that are FDA approved specifically to treat hypoactive sexual desire disorder are:

Flibanserin (Addyi®) and bremelanotide (VyleesiTM). Both are only approved for (presumably cis) women who are not yet entering menopause. Addyi made a big splash when it was approved in 2015 (and relaunched in 2018 at a lower price point because it didn't do fantastically) for low sex drive that was acquired (wasn't always as low as it is now) and generalized (meaning not related to having a a stressful or crappy relationship with one person).

Media fluffed it as a 'female viagra' though it is meant to increase sexual desire and doesn't do anything for blood flow like Viagra. The best clinical trial found that Addyi increased sexual events to .5 to 1 more event per month. Addyi has had some continuing concerns since it's been on the market and at the time of me writing this (late 2021) is being evaluated by the Food and Drug Administration for regulatory action for inducing drug hypersensitivity.

Vyleesi (bremelanotide) dropped in 2019, as an injectible pre-sex alternative. It's a shot you take 45 minutes before sexitimes is expected, in order to stimulate melanocortin-4 receptors. Melanocortin is a hormone that is tied to our social and sexual behaviors. Research shows that Vyleesi does not interfere with hormonal birth controls and you can still have a glass of wine while using it. 8% of individuals in a 6 month study experienced increased desire as a result of the medication.

This probably all makes it sound like I am categorically anti-Addyi and anti-Vyleesi. I'm not. I'm anti billionaire-privatizing-space-travel, but unlike that bullshit, these medications have created some positive change in some people's lives, even if it's incremental. Do keep in mind that you may not have great insurance coverage on these drugs. Even though ED medications are also "lifestyle" medications, they are far more likely to be covered by insurance if you have a penis than these medications will be covered if you have a vulva. Once again hitting the idea that our sexual response is not a problem that needs solving.

One final possibility is the O-Shot®. This is a platelet-rich plasma (PRP) made from the patient's own blood. This is not an FDA approved treatment, because the FDA doesn't govern blood biologics (though the process for producing the PRP is used with FDA approved equipment). The shot was created by Dr. Charles Runels based on the research that shows that PRP stimulates stem cells, collagen production, and blood vessels which is used for healing injuries elsewhere in the body, with the hope that it would stimulate more blood flow and nerve generation throughout the glans, labia, and internal parts of the clitoris… which could lead to better orgasms and sex in the women he studied.

Runels completed one pilot study in 2014 with positive outcomes (71% of the 11 women in the study went from "distressed" to "not distressed") and there has been other anecdotal data reported around the world since. This one will definitely be an out-of-pocket treatment unless you have some ballin' insurance plan that I've never heard of.

I've had multiple clients try many varieties of these treatments over the years and have heard positive feedback on a lot of them. While none of these are as easy-peasy a fix as popping a blood flow pill for a penis, we are finally starting to get some options on the market.

SURGICAL OPTIONS

Sometimes, though, there are issues that are physical, not biochemical, which means that surgical options may make more sense.

Clitoral hood reduction

Imagine how painful it would be if all 8000 nerve endings of the clitoral glans were out exposed all the time, rubbing against your clothes constantly (and not in a fun way). The hood over the clitoris offers protection of the area and is clearly a necessary feature. However some people have extra skin in that area which gets in the way of accessing the glans when we want those nerves stimulated. Having some of the skin reduced is an out-of-pocket (it's considered cosmetic, once again, though we all are in agreement that's bullshit) in office procedure that some people opt for and have found beneficial.

Hood reduction

BEFORE

AFTER

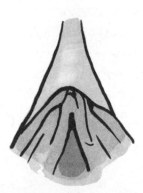 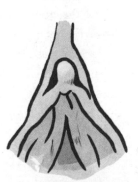

CLITORAL RECONSTRUCTION

The World Health Organization (WHO) estimates that 200 million individuals with vulvae are living with female genital mutilation/cutting (FGM/C). FGM/C is the partial or total removal of the external glans of the clitoris for cultural/religious reasons.

WHO estimates that it continues to be inflicted upon another 3 million individuals a year (and UNICEF estimates more than 4 million). We think of this as being something rare when it clearly is no such thing, and happens all over the world, not just in developing nations.

Surgical interventions on intersex infants (which was the go-to treatment modality for many decades and still happens way too fucking often) can also cause scarring, issues with sensation, incontinence, etc., as well.

Along with the loss of glans, there have also been many cases of nerve tumors (traumatic neuromas) growing where the nerves were lesioned which creates incredible neuropathic pain which also requires surgical intervention.

Remember the bad-ass docs who fully mapped the internal structure of the clitoris a few years ago? They are surgeons who specialize in clitoral reconstruction after FGM/C. It's a new surgery that we only know is feasible because of our newly-acquired knowledge about the complexity of the clitoral structure. Data on safety and outcomes is still limited, but you may be able to reduce pain, match pre-mutilation appearance, and increase pleasure.

STI PREVENTION AND SAFETY

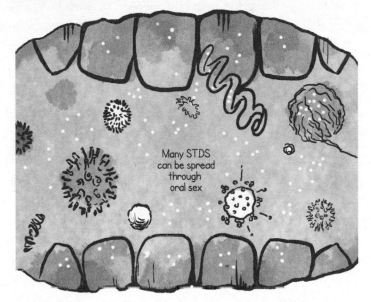

Many STDS can be spread through oral sex

s oral sex generally safer than penetrative intercourse? Absolutely. Can you still transmit STIs through oral sex? Also absolutely. And that includes:

- Chlamydia
- Gonorrhea
- Syphilis
- Herpes
- HPV (human papillomavirus)
- HIV

Firstly, whether using barrier protection or not, don't brush your teeth for two hours before or two hours after oral sex. While your attention to oral hygiene is deeply appreciated, keep to a nice mouthwash gargle, because brushing does create bleeding gums and microabrasions in most of us, and that becomes an entry point for all kinds of cooties.

Now for barrier methods? There is plenty of stuff on the market to help with that. Condoms aren't flavored because vaginas, penises, and anuses like the taste of strawberry!

Along with condoms (both internal and external), we have gloves and finger cots (which can be specifically helpful for oral sex after metoidioplasty), and sex dams. Additionally, a Malaysian gynecologist recently released a condom created from adhesive surgical dressing that can be used in a multitude of ways (innies, outies, and all aroundies). If you are not in a closed relationship where everyone has been given the all-clear, or have been tested with certain partners and agreed to use barrier protection with others, please please please glove your love. And consider both a pre-exposure prophylaxis (PrEP) to way reduce your risk of getting HIV and post-exposure prophylaxis (PEP) if you aren't taking PrEP and you have a barrier method failure during sexitimes.

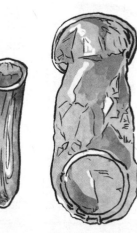

One hack that Auntie is cool with? While condoms cannot be DIY'd, sex dams can! Condoms can be cut open (and while you don't want to use a sperimicidal condom for oral sex, you can use one for a dam conversion, so long as the spericidal part isn't where your mouth is going).

Disposable gloves (which make manual sex safer on its own) can also be converted into a dam by cutting off the fingers and then cutting open the palm of the glove along one side and unfolding it. But even easier? Saran Wrap as a barrier dam has proven to be effective in the prevention of the spread of STIs. Super easy.

Another trick I picked up from the Scarleteen website about sex dams is to write a non-reversible letter, number, or symbol on one side of the dam so you don't accidentally reverse the dam later during play.

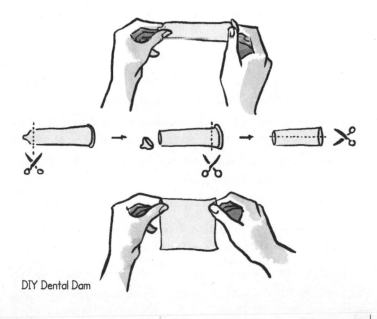

DIY Dental Dam

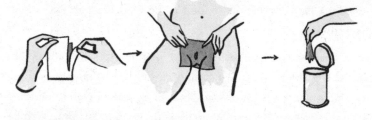

Dental dam
(used on vagina and anus)

Clean Your Toys Properly

I know, I know...the whole point of having toys is so that you DON'T have to use barrier methods to prevent pregnancy and STIs. But while a toy won't get you pregnant, you can still pass on STIs through toys that were not properly cleaned (not just to and from other people, but even reinfecting yourself with something that had already been treated).

Whether DIY or one you purchased, take good care of your goodies! Don't use a perfumed soap, the ingredients used for scent can irritate your skin. Dr. Bronner's soap is great stuff and comes unscented for sensitive folx. A good quality antibacterial soap is best. You want to wipe them down, not dunk them (unless they are a waterproof toy then dunk away).

Don't put your rubber and plastic type toys in the dishwasher, you can totally melt them. Other than glass toys or stainless steel, you wanna stay away from the dishwasher.

Leather—Wipe down with soap and water or use a special leather cleaner. If the leather comes in contact with bodily fluids, you can disinfect it by wiping it down with a 70% isopropyl rubbing alcohol solution.

Glass—Wash with soap and water

Rubber—if it's something that is going to be inserted, use a condom or dam (see below)...rubber is super porous so they hold bacterial grubbies way too well. Also? Rubber can contain phthalate, which is not something you want seeping into your never-minds (if you wouldn't eat it, don't stick it up anywhere, either).

Silicone—Wash with soap and water

Stainless steel—Wash with soap and water. If you want to be extra about it, stainless steel can go in the dishwasher or can be soaked in a solution of 10:1 water and bleach for ten minutes.

Vinyl and Cyberskin—These are very porous materials that are pretty fragile. These are best washed in warm water and air dried. They can get sticky easily so dusting them with cornstarch is also a good idea (fun fact: corn starch doesn't clump up).

Nylon (paracord is made of nylon, FYI)—Can be washed in the washing machine or by hand with soap and water. You can also remove odor from nylon by soaking it in a solution of water and baking soda.

Fabrics—Wash all fabric as you would fabric you are wearing on your body. Cotton, polyester, and bamboo and the like does fine in a washing machine, silks and wools do better dry cleaned or gently hand washed if you feel confident in managing these materials. Fabric ropes need to be left to be air dried in coils and and stretched occasionally during the drying period so they don't kink up (you are already kinky enough, right, playa?)

Hemp—Hemp can be machine washed on gentle and air dried (it will take 2-5 days to dry completely, so plan accordingly). If you are washing hemp rope, you will want to knot it and and place it in a pillow case before washing (there are lots of videos online with knotting techniques to prepare rope for washing). Hemp rope can be reoiled (baby oil or jojoba oil are good) after drying)

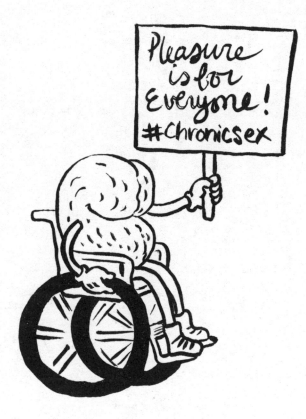

CONCLUSION

Y'all. Y'all? Too much time sitting here trying to figure out how one concludes a book on oral sex. I could make some terrible dad jokes (but already did that).

I could be cheerfully encouraging of you getting down with any oral pleasure your heart desires (but already did that, too). And anytime I write anything really insightful and cool in a conclusion, my editor ends up moving it somewhere else in the book and making a whole new conclusion.

Which means I kinda can't win. And yet, this book doesn't go to print without a conclusion (tried that, too).

So I'm going to go with a "thank you" conclusion. I'm writing this last bit after we launched the pre-order and the response has been amazing. So many people are hungry for books of this nature that are practical and comprehensive and full of geekery-science fun. And I deeply appreciate that you trust me with providing that content to you. I talked earlier in this book about culture being anything we create. And I'm so proud of this empowered and inclusive world we are creating together.

See you again soon!

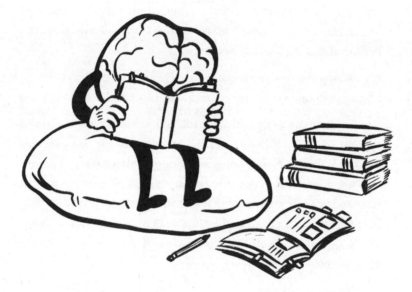

REFERENCES

8 things to know about sex and her period. Men's Journal. (2021, May 29). Retrieved November 30, 2021, from mensjournal.com/health-fitness/8-things-every-man-should-know-about-sex-and-her-period-20151216/.

Abdulcadir, J., Rodriguez, M. I., Petignat, P., & Say, L. (2015). Clitoral reconstruction after female genital mutilation/cutting: case studies. The journal of sexual medicine, 12(1), 274–281. https://doi.org/10.1111/jsm.12737

Abdulcadir, J., Tille, J. C., & Petignat, P. (2017). Management of painful clitoral neuroma after female genital mutilation/cutting. Reproductive health, 14(1), 22. https://doi.org/10.1186/s12978-017-0288-3

Addyi explained: It's use in hypoactive sexual desire disorder. Drugs.com. (n.d.). Retrieved December 13, 2021, from drugs.com/slideshow/addyi-explained-1202.

All That's Interesting. (2019, July 31). A photographic history of the Dildo, one of humanity's most enduring tools. All That's Interesting. Retrieved September 23, 2021, from https://allthatsinteresting.com/history-of-the-dildo.

A period sex guide for Queer Women & People with vulvas. Daye. (n.d.). Retrieved November 30, 2021, from https://yourdaye.com/vitals/womens-health/period-sex-guide-for-queer-women.

Aswell, S. (2018, August 22). *Learn more about your clitoris: It's not just a tiny nub.* Healthline. Retrieved November 29, 2021, from healthline.com/health/womens-health/clitoris-like-an-iceberg-for-pleasure#Keep-the-learning-inside-and-out.

Banmen, J. (2002). The Satir Model: Yesterday and Today. Contemporary Family Therapy, 24(1), 7-22.

Bansal AS, Chee R, Nagendran V, Warner A, & Hayman G (2007). Dangerous liaison: sexually transmitted allergic reaction to Brazil nuts. Journal of investigational allergology & clinical immunology : official organ of the International Association of Asthmology (INTERASMA) and Sociedad Latinoamericana de Alergia e Inmunologia, 17 (3), 189-91 PMID: 17583107

Basson, . (2005). Women's sexual dysfunction: Revised and expanded definitions. CMAJ : Canadian Medical Association journal = journal de l'Association medicale canadienne. 172. 1327-33. 10.1503/cmaj.1020174.

Basson R. (2010). Testosterone therapy for reduced libido in women. *Therapeutic advances in endocrinology and metabolism*, 1(4), 155–164. https://doi.org/10.1177/2042018810379588

Berman, L., Berman, J., Miles, M., Pollets, D., & Powell, J. A. (2003). Genital self-image as a component of sexual health: relationship between genital self-image, female sexual function, and quality of life measures. Journal of sex & marital therapy, 29 Suppl 1, 11–21. https://doi.org/10.1080/713847124

Blair, K. L., Cappell, J., & Pukall, C. F. (2017). Not all orgasms were created equal: Differences in frequency and satisfaction of orgasm experiences by sexual activity in same-sex versus mixed-sex relationships. The Journal of Sex Research, 55(6), 719–733. https://doi.org/10.1080/00224499.2017.1303437

Blank, J., & Corinne, T. (2011). Femalia. Last Gasp.

Braswell, S. (2015). How the mob introduced Americans to oral sex. Yahoo! Sports. Retrieved October 7, 2021, from http://sports.yahoo.com/news/mob-introduced-americans-oral-sex-080000538.html.

Brice, R. (2019, August 1). U up? how does HRT affect your sex and libido? Healthline. Retrieved October 14, 2021, from healthline.com/health/healthy-sex/hrt-sexuality-libido#4.

Bonham, K. (2013, October 30). *Sexually Transmitted Food allergens*. Scientific American Blog Network. Retrieved November 23, 2021, from https://blogs.scientificamerican.com/food-matters/sexually-transmitted-food-allergens/.

Callen-Lorde. (2021). Pump: Sexual Pleasure & Health Resource Guide for Transmen who

have Sex with Men. Retrieved October 14, 2021, from http://callen-lorde.org/graphics/2021/02/PUMP-TMSM-Health-Guide_Final_V3.2.pdf

Campbell, J. (2020, July 29). Everything we should've grown up knowing about Intersexuality. Volonté. Retrieved October 14, 2021, from lelo.com/blog/intersexuality/.

Center for Drug Evaluation and Research. (n.d.). January - March 2021: Potential Signals of serious risks/new safety. U.S. Food and Drug Administration. Retrieved November 29, 2021, from fda.gov/drugs/questions-and-answers-fdas-adverse-event-reporting-system-faers/january-march-2021-potential-signals-serious-risksnew-safety-information-identified-fda-adverse.

Centers for Disease Control and Prevention. (2020, September 16). *Disability impacts all of us infographic*. Centers for Disease Control and Prevention. Retrieved November 16, 2021, from cdc.gov/ncbddd/disabilityandhealth/infographic-disability-impacts-all.html#:%7E:text=61%E2%80%8Amillion%E2%80%8Aadults%E2%80%8Ain%E2%80%8Athe%2Chave%E2%80%8Asome%E2%80%8Atype%E2%80%8Aof%E2%80%8Adisability.

Centers for Disease Control and Prevention. (2020, September 16). *Disability and health overview*. Centers for Disease Control and Prevention. Retrieved November 16, 2021, from cdc.gov/ncbddd/disabilityandhealth/disability.html.

Center for Women's Health. OHSU. (n.d.). Retrieved October 14, 2021, from ohsu.edu/womens-health/benefits-healthy-sex-life.

Chen, A. (2020, September 9). What brain scans tell us about sex. maude. Retrieved October 14, 2021, from https://getmaude.com/blogs/themaudern/on-what-brain-scans-can-tell-us-about-sex.

Cirino, E. (2019, November 24). The O-shot and PRP: What it is, uses, research, and more. Healthline. Retrieved November 29, 2021, from healthline.com/health/o-shot#uses-and-research.

Clitoral hood reduction Houston, TX. Memorial Plastic Surgery. Retrieved December 13, 2021, from memorialplasticsurgery.com/clitoral-hood-reduction-houston-texas/.

Cohen, J. (2021, July 15). Female sexual dysfunction drug addyi faces yet another setback. Forbes. Retrieved November 29, 2021, from forbes.com/sites/joshuacohen/2021/07/15/female-sexual-dysfunction-drug-addyi-faces-yet-another-setback/?sh=2df4c47ad175.

Cunnilingus and menstruation?: GO ASK Alice! dummy image. (n.d.). Retrieved November 30, 2021, from https://goaskalice.columbia.edu/answered-questions/cunnilingus-and-menstruation.

Female genital mutilation (FGM) statistics. UNICEF DATA. (2021, September 10). Retrieved December 13, 2021, from https://data.unicef.org/topic/child-protection/female-genital-mutilation/.

Female genital mutilation. UNICEF. (2020, February 5). Retrieved December 13, 2021, from unicef.org/protection/female-genital-mutilation.

Fellizar, K. (2021, May 25). 12 guys share what oral sex really feels like for them. Bustle. Retrieved October 13, 2021, from bustle.com/wellness/90841-what-do-blow-jobs-feel-like-for-men-12-men-share-what-they-really-think-of.

Foldes, P., & Buisson, O. (2009). The clitoral complex: a dynamic sonographic study. The journal of sexual medicine, 6(5), 1223–1231. https://doi.org/10.1111/j.1743-6109.2009.01231.x

Foreplay. Foreplay - an overview | ScienceDirect Topics. (n.d.). Retrieved October 13, 2021, from sciencedirect.com/topics/medicine-and-dentistry/foreplay.

Fredrick, D. (2002). The Roman Gaze Vision, power and the body. The Johns Hopkins University Press.

Freeman S (1986). Woman allergic to husband's sweat and semen. Contact dermatitis, 14 (2), 110-2 PMID: 3709144

Glamour. (2016, June 16). Does what you eat affect how your vagina tastes? SELF. Retrieved January 19, 2022, from self.com/story/what-you-eat-affect-vagina-tastes

González, M., Viáfara, G., Caba, F., & Molina, E. (2004). Sexual function, menopause and hormone replacement therapy (HRT). *Maturitas*, 48(4), 411–420. https://doi.org/10.1016/j.maturitas.2003.10.005

Good, giving, and game: Research confirms that Dan Savage's sex advice works. PsyPost. (2015, April 16). Retrieved September 24, 2021, from psypost.org/2014/10/good-giving-game-research-confirms-dan-savages-sex-advice-works-28965.

Gurza, A. (2016, September 22). Deepthroating while disabled: The symbolism, realities and importance of oral sex to the Queer Cripple. HuffPost. Retrieved September 29, 2021, from huffpost.com/entry/deepthroating-while-disabled-the-symbolism-realities_b_57e3fc80e4b05d3737be5674.

Haber, R. (2002). Virginia Satir: An Integrated, Humanistic Approach. Contemporary

Family Therapy, 24(1), 23-34.

Herbenick, D., & Reece, M. (2010). Development and validation of the female genital self-image scale. The journal of sexual medicine, 7(5), 1822–1830. https://doi.org/10.1111/j.1743-6109.2010.01728.x

Hitchens, C. (2006, October 10). As American as Apple Pie. Vanity Fair. Retrieved October 13, 2021, from vanityfair.com/news/2006/07/hitchens200607.

Hitti, M. (2006, February 22). Men's sex lives better at 50 than 30. WebMD. Retrieved October 20, 2021, from webmd.com/men/news/20060222/mens-sex-lives-better-50-than-30.

hollowc2. (2020, September 4). *There's help for women who can't achieve orgasm*. Cleveland Clinic. Retrieved November 28, 2021, from https://health.clevelandclinic.org/theres-help-for-women-who-cant-achieve-orgasm/.

How to eat out a non-op trans woman. VICE. (n.d.). Retrieved October 14, 2021, from vice.com/en/article/594mak/how-to-eat-out-a-non-op-trans-woman-oral-sex.

How to have a healthy sex life: What to know about orgasms, safety, and your brain. theSkimm. (n.d.). Retrieved October 13, 2021, from theskimm.com/well/healthy-sex-life-guide-WqmsyJtUmknZpUrEAcBIC?utm_source=newsletter_ds&utm_medium=email.

Infographic: Sexual behavior in the United States Today. Sex and Psychology. (2021, October 7). Retrieved November 28, 2021, from sexandpsychology.com/blog/2016/1/13/infographic-sexual-behavior-in-the-united-states-today/.

"I want to be like nature made me". Human Rights Watch. (2020, December 15). Retrieved November 29, 2021, from hrw.org/report/2017/07/25/i-want-be-nature-made-me/medically-unnecessary-surgeries-intersex-children-us.

Jewell, T. (2019, January 10). DHT: How it causes hair loss and how to slow it. Healthline. Retrieved December 10, 2021, from healthline.com/health/dht.

Jozkowski KN, Herbenick D, Schick V, Reece M, Sanders SA, Fortenberry JD. Women's perceptions about lubricant use and vaginal wetness during sexual activities. The Journal of Sexual Medicine. 2013 Feb 1;10(2):484–92

Kilchevsky, A., Vardi, Y., Lowenstein, L., & Gruenwald, I. (2012). Is the female G-spot truly a distinct anatomic entity?. The journal of sexual medicine, 9(3), 719–726. https://doi.org/10.1111/j.1743-6109.2011.02623.x

Kirakosyan, D. A., About The Author Armen Kirakosyan, & Kirakosyan, A. (2019, April 18). *Is clitoral hood reduction surgery the right step for you?* Aesthetic Gynecology Specialists of WNY. Retrieved December 13, 2021, from aestheticgynecologyofwny.com/blog/is-clitoral-hood-reduction-surgery-the-right-step-for-you-cost-and-benefits.

Klein, C., & Gorzalka, B. B. (2009). Sexual functioning in transsexuals following hormone therapy and genital surgery: a review. The journal of sexual medicine, 6(11), 2922–2941. https://doi.org/10.1111/j.1743-6109.2009.01370.x

Knapp, H. (2006). Pornography - The Secret History of Civilisation [DVD]. United ingdom; Koch Vision.

Kovalevsky G. (2005). Female sexual dysfunction and use of hormone therapy in postmenopausal women. Seminars in reproductive medicine, 23(2), 180–187. https://doi.org/10.1055/s-2005-869486

Lastella, M., O'Mullan, C., Paterson, J. L., & Reynolds, A. C. (2019). Sex and Sleep: Perceptions of Sex as a Sleep Promoting Behavior in the General Adult Population. Frontiers in public health, 7, 33. https://doi.org/10.3389/fpubh.2019.00033

Lee, B. Y. (2019, March 13). Why a woman suffered an allergic reaction from oral sex. Forbes. Retrieved November 23, 2021, from forbes.com/sites/brucelee/2019/03/12/why-a-woman-had-an-allergic-reaction-after-oral-sex/?sh=4d0e69f341da.

Levin RJ. VIP, vagina, clitoral and periurethral glans—an update on human female genital arousal. Experimental and Clinical Endocrinology & Diabetes. 1991;98(05):61–9.

Levin RJ. The physiology of sexual arousal in the human female: a recreational and procreational synthesis. Archives of Sexual Behavior. 2002 Oct 1;31(5):405–11.

Ley, D. J. (2016). Ethical porn for dicks: A man's guide to responsible viewing pleasure. ThreeL Media.

Lister, K. (2020, July 17). *A brief history of oral sex, from ancient China to DJ Khaled*. inews.co.uk. Retrieved November 28, 2021, from https://inews.co.uk/opinion/comment/a-brief-history-of-oral-sex-from-ancient-china-to-dj-khaled-152919.

Little, C. (2021, October 12). Your partner can totally go down on you during your period (& it can even help with cramps). SheKnows. Retrieved November 30, 2021, from sheknows.com/health-and-wellness/articles/1131608/yes-your-partner-can-go-down-on-you-during-your-period/.

Liu, H., Shen, S., & Hsieh, N. (2019). A National Dyadic Study of Oral Sex, Relationship Quality, and Well-Being among Older Couples. The journals of gerontology. Series B, Psychological sciences and social sciences, 74(2), 298–308. https://doi.org/10.1093/geronb/gby089

Liu, H., Shen, S., & Hsieh, N. (2018). ORAL SEX FOR OLDER LOVERS: IMPLICATIONS ON RELATIONSHIP QUALITY AND MENTAL HEALTH. Innovation in Aging, 2(Suppl 1), 583. https://doi.org/10.1093/geroni/igy023.2162

Liu, H., Shen, S., & Hsieh, N. (2019, February 20). Oral sex is good for older couples. OUPblog. Retrieved September 29, 2021, from https://blog.oup.com/2019/02/oral-sex-older-couples/.

MailOnline, V. W. for. (2015, January 14). 'Sex toys' dating back 28,000 years made from stone and dried camel dung. Daily Mail Online. Retrieved September 24, 2021, from dailymail.co.uk/sciencetech/article-2908415/The-sex-toys-dating-28-000-years-Ancient-phalluses-stone-dried-camel-dung-started-trend-sex-aids.html.

Manske, M. (2019, October 4). Circular breathing: Uses, benefits, and how to master the technique. Healthline. Retrieved December 6, 2021, from healthline.com/health/circular-breathing#for-instruments.

Marchione, M. (2007, August 22). Sex and the seniors: Survey shows many elderly people remain frisky. The New York Times. Retrieved September 29, 2021, from nytimes.com/2007/08/22/health/22iht-22sex.7216942.html.

Marin, V. (2019, January 24). Why oral sex can trigger anxiety for people with PTSD. Allure. Retrieved October 21, 2021, from allure.com/story/oral-sex-anxiety-after-sexual-assault.

Mayo Foundation for Medical Education and Research. (2020, April 4). Allergy skin tests. Mayo Clinic. Retrieved December 9, 2021, from mayoclinic.org/tests-procedures/allergy-tests/about/pac-20392895#:~:text=Patch%20tests%20can%20detect%20delayed,that%20can%20cause%20contact%20dermatitis.

McCabe, M. P., & Taleporos, G. (2003). Sexual esteem, sexual satisfaction, and sexual behavior among people with physical disability. Archives of sexual behavior, 32(4), 359–369. https://doi.org/10.1023/a:1024047100251

Midori. (2018, November 29). Oral success. Men's Health. Retrieved December 1, 2021, from menshealth.com/uk/sex/a745099/mh-masterclass-oral-sex-26889/.

Miller, K. (2021, November 2). There's a chance that oral sex could feel even better on your period, experts say. Women's Health. Retrieved November 30, 2021, from womenshealthmag.com/sex-and-love/a19966800/oral-sex-on-period/.

Mitrokostas, B. I. (n.d.). *Here's what happens to your body and Brain when you orgasm*. ScienceAlert. Retrieved November 19, 2021, from sciencealert.com/here-s-what-happens-to-your-brain-when-you-orgasm.

Moon, A. (2020). Getting it. Potter/Ten Speed/Harmony/Rodale.

Moore, A. (2021, June 24). All vaginas are different: Here are 9 different ways it can look, from OB/Gyns. mindbodygreen. Retrieved January 19, 2022, from mindbodygreen.com/articles/types-of-vaginas

Mota R. L. (2017). Female urinary incontinence and sexuality. International braz j urol : official journal of the Brazilian Society of Urology, 43(1), 20–28. https://doi.org/10.1590/S1677-5538.IBJU.2016.0102

Muise, A., & Impett, E. A. (2016). Applying theories of communal motivation to sexuality. Social and Personality Psychology Compass, 10(8), 455–467. https://doi.org/10.1111/spc3.12261

Muise, A., & Impett, E. A. (2014). Good, giving, and Game. Social Psychological and Personality Science, 6(2), 164–172. https://doi.org/10.1177/1948550614553641

Nature Publishing Group. (n.d.). Nature news. Retrieved October 20, 2021, from nature.com/scitable/blog/brain-metrics/what_does_fmri_measure/.

O'Connor, M. (2014, September 16). Blood hounds: They're obsessed with period sex. The Cut. Retrieved November 30, 2021, from thecut.com/2014/09/blood-hounds-theyre-obsessed-with-period-sex.html.

O-shot® safety. Coyle Institute. (2021, July 29). Retrieved December 13, 2021, from https://coyleinstitute.com/o-shot-safety/.

Pantozzi, J., (2012, January 17). We discovered the clitoris in 2009? heyyy, wait a minute... The Mary Sue. Retrieved November 29, 2021, from themarysue.com/clitoris-discovery-2009/.

Post-traumatic stress, sexual trauma and dissociative ... (n.d.). Retrieved October 21, 2021, from ojp.gov/pdffiles1/Photocopy/153416NCJRS.pdf.

Potenza M. N. (2013). Neurobiology of gambling behaviors. Current opinion in neurobiology, 23(4), 660–667. https://doi.org/10.1016/j.conb.2013.03.004

Puppo, V., & Gruenwald, I. (2012). Does the G-spot exist? A review of the current literature. International urogynecology journal, 23(12), 1665–1669. https://doi.org/10.1007/s00192-012-1831-y

Rodden, J. (2020, October 8). These medications cause low libido. The Checkup. Retrieved October 20, 2021, from singlecare.com/blog/low-libido-caused-by-medication/

Romm, C. (2018, May 9). 11 sex therapists on what their clients tell them about oral sex. The Cut. Retrieved November 28, 2021, from thecut.com/2018/05/11-sex-therapists-on-what-their-clients-say-about-oral-sex.html.

Ross, C., & Dodson, B. (2017). Betty Dodson Bodysex basics. Betty A. Dodson Foundation.

Rubio-Casillas, A., & Jannini, E. A. (2011). New insights from one case of female ejaculation. The Journal of Sexual Medicine, 8(12), 3500–3504. https://doi.org/10.1111/j.1743-6109.2011.02472.x

Runels, C. (2014). A pilot study of the effect of localized injections of autologous platelet rich plasma (PRP) for the treatment of female sexual dysfunction. Journal of Women's Health Care, 03(04). https://doi.org/10.4172/2167-0420.1000169

Russell, T. (2011). A renegade history of the United States. Free Press.

Salama, S., Boitrelle, F., Gauquelin, A., Malagrida, L., Thiounn, N., & Desvaux, P. (2015). Nature and origin of "squirting" in female sexuality. The journal of sexual medicine, 12(3), 661–666. https://doi.org/10.1111/jsm.12799

Santos-Longhurst, A. (2019, November 12). 15 faqs about female ejaculation. Healthline. Retrieved November 29, 2021, from healthline.com/health/healthy-sex/female-ejaculation#urine-and-ejaculate.

Sayles, C. (2002). Transformational Change – based on the Model of Virginia Satir.

Contemporary Family Therapy, 24(1), 93-109.

Schiotz, H.A., Bohlin, T. Klingen, T.A., and Aaberg, T. "Neuroma in the clitoris after circumcision," Journal of the Norwegian Medical Association, vol. 6, no. 132, pp. 629-630, 2012.

Sovetkina, E., Weiss, M., & Verplanken, B. (2017). Perception of vulnerability in young females' experiences of oral sex: Findings from the focus group discussions. Cogent Psychology, 4(1), 1418643. https://doi.org/10.1080/23311908.2017.1418643

Stis: Ways to make sex safer. Region of Peel - Working for you. (n.d.). Retrieved December 6, 2021, from peelregion.ca/health/sexuality/sti/comm-safe.htm.

Stoya. (2019, September 17). I refuse oral sex from guys for a very good reason. do I owe them an explanation? Slate Magazine. Retrieved October 21, 2021, from https://slate.com/human-interest/2019/09/sex-act-panic-attacks-explanation-sex-advice.html.

Swartz, A. (2021, May 27). A history of oral sex, from Fellatio's ancient roots to the modern blow job. Mic. Retrieved September 24, 2021, from mic.

com/p/a-history-of-oral-sex-from-fellatios-ancient-roots-to-the-modern-blow-job-16543812.

Sweeney, E. (2016, June 23). Getting and giving head when you're disabled. Wear Your Voice. Retrieved September 29, 2021, from wearyourvoicemag. com/tips-oral-sex-youre-disabled/.

Testosterone HRT & Bottom Growth. FOLX Health. (n.d.). Retrieved December 10, 2021, from https://folxhealth.com/library/testosterone-bottom-growth.

The clitoris was only fully discovered in 1998. babe. (2017, May 25). Retrieved December 6, 2021, from https://babe.net/2017/02/02/clitoris-fully-discovered-1998-650.

The Irish Times. (2017, January 23). The clitoris has 8,000 nerve endings (and nine other things we learned from a new artwork). The Irish Times. Retrieved December 6, 2021, from irishtimes.com/life-and-style/health-family/the-clitoris-has-8-000-nerve-endings-and-nine-other-things-we-learned-from-a-new-artwork-1.2947694.

Troeller, L., & Schneider, M. (2014). Orgasm: Photographs & interviews. Daylight.

Vaginoplasty: Procedure details, risks, benefits & recovery. Cleveland Clinic. (n.d.). Retrieved November 29, 2021, from https://my.clevelandclinic. org/health/treatments/21572-vaginoplasty.

Vulture. (2008, March 17). How dirty is that Auden poem that was too dirty for the 'times book review'? Vulture. Retrieved October 13, 2021, from vulture.com/2008/03/how_dirty_is_that_auden_poem_t.html.

Vyleesi fact sheet: National women's health network. National Women's Health Network |. (2021, April 10). Retrieved December 13, 2021, from https://nwhn. org/vyleesi-fact-sheet/.

Waite, L. J., Laumann, E. O., Das, A., & Schumm, L. P. (2009). Sexuality: measures of partnerships, practices, attitudes, and problems in the National Social Life, Health, and Aging Study. The journals of gerontology. Series B, Psychological sciences and social sciences, 64 Suppl 1(Suppl 1), i56–i66. https:// doi.org/10.1093/geronb/gbp038

Weiss, S. (2016, May 24). Scientists explain the weird reason why we have oral sex. Glamour. Retrieved October 13, 2021, from glamour.com/story/ why-we-have-oral-sex.

Whipple, B., & Komisaruk, B. R. (1985). Elevation of pain threshold by vaginal stimulation in women. Pain, 21(4), 357–367. https://doi.org/10.1016/0304-3959(85)90164-2

Wickman, D. (2017). 232 plasticity of the skene's gland in women who report fluid ejaculation with orgasm. The Journal of Sexual Medicine, 14(1). https://doi.org/10.1016/j.jsxm.2016.11.147

Wise, N. J., Frangos, E., & Komisaruk, B. R. (2017). Brain activity unique to orgasm in women: An fmri analysis. The Journal of Sexual Medicine, 14(11), 1380–1391. https://doi.org/10.1016/j.jsxm.2017.08.014

Wimpissinger, F., Springer, C., & Stackl, W. (2013). International online survey: Female Ejaculation has a positive impact on women's and their partners' sexual lives. BJU International, 112(2). https://doi.org/10.1111/j.1464-410x.2012.11562.x

Wood, J. R., McKay, A., Komarnicky, T., & Milhausen, R. R. (2016). Was it good for you too?: An analysis of gender differences in oral sex practices and pleasure ratings among heterosexual Canadian university students. The Canadian Journal of Human Sexuality, 25(1), 21–29. https://doi.org/10.3138/cjhs.251-a2

World Health Organization. (n.d.). Female genital mutilation. World Health Organization. Retrieved December 13, 2021, from who.int/newsroom/fact-sheets/detail/female-genital-mutilation#:~:text=More%20than%203%20million%20girls,countries%20where%20population%20data%20exist.

Wright, H., Jenks, R. A., Demeyere, N. Frequent Sexual Activity Predicts Specific Cognitive Abilities in Older Adults, The Journals of Gerontology: Series B, Volume 74, Issue 1, January 2019, Pages 47–51, https://doi.org/10.1093/geronb/gbx065

ABOUT THE AUTHOR

Faith Harper PhD, LPC-S, ACS, ACN is a bad-ass, funny lady with a PhD. She's a licensed professional counselor, board supervisor, certified sexologist, and applied clinical nutritionist with a private practice and consulting business in San Antonio, TX. She has been an adjunct professor and a TEDx presenter, and proudly identifies as a woman of color and uppity intersectional feminist. She is the author of dozens of books.

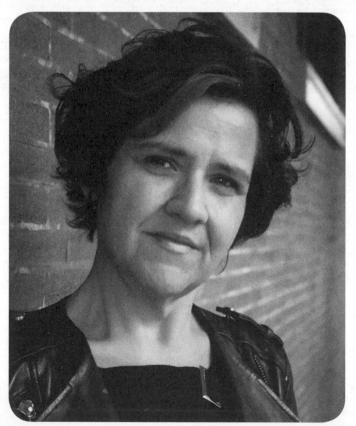

MORE BY DR. FAITH

Books
The Autism Relationships Handbook (with Joe Biel)
Befriend Your Brain
Coping Skills
How to Be Accountable (with Joe Biel)
This Is Your Brain on Depression
Unfuck Your Addiction (with Joseph E Green)
Unfuck Your Adulting
Unfuck Your Anger
Unfuck Your Anxiety
Unfuck Your Blow Jobs
Unfuck Your Body
Unfuck Your Boundaries
Unfuck Your Brain
Unfuck Your Cunnilingus
Unfuck Your Friendships
Unfuck Your Grief
Unfuck Your Intimacy
Unfuck Your Worth
Unfuck Your Writing (with Joe Biel)
Woke Parenting (with Bonnie Scott)

Workbooks
Achieve Your Goals
The Autism Relationships Workbook (with Joe Biel)
How to Be Accountable Workbook (with Joe Biel)
Unfuck Your Anger Workbook
Unfuck Your Anxiety Workbook
Unfuck Your Body Workbook
Unfuck Your Boundaries Workbook
Unfuck Your Intimacy Workbook
Unfuck Your Worth Workbook
Unfuck Your Year

Zines
The Autism Handbook (with Joe Biel)
The Autism Partner Handbook (with Joe Biel)
BDSM FAQ
Dating
Defriending
Detox Your Masculinity (with Aaron Sapp)
Emotional Freedom Technique
Getting Over It
How to Find a Therapist
How to Say No
Indigenous Noms
Relationshipping
The Revolution Won't Forget the Holidays
Self-Compassion
Sex Tools
Sexing Yourself
STI FAQ (with Aaron Sapp)
Surviving
This Is Your Brain on Addiction
This Is Your Brain on Grief
This Is Your Brain on PTSD
Unfuck Your Consent
Unfuck Your Forgiveness
Unfuck Your Mental Health Paradigm
Unfuck Your Sleep
Unfuck Your Work
Vision Boarding
Woke Parenting #1-6 (with Bonnie Scott)

Other
Boundaries Conversation Deck
How Do You Feel Today? (poster)

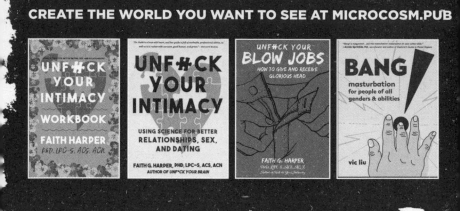
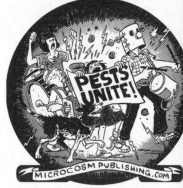
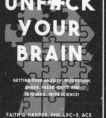
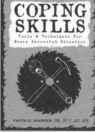
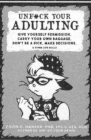
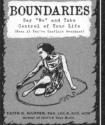
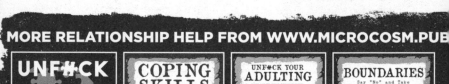